The Book About,
IT

The Book About, IT

ME AND YOU AGAINST THE WORLD

AN AUTOBIOGRAPHY OF AND BY:

CYNTHIA MARIE

A Cynthia Marie yes that's me! Book inc.
on the subject of
Gender//Dysphoria

iUniverse, Inc.
Bloomington

The Book About, IT:
Me And You Against the World

iUniverse books may be ordered through booksellers or by contacting:

iUniverse
1663 Liberty Drive
Bloomington, IN 47403
www.iuniverse.com
1-800-Authors (1-800-288-4677)

ISBN: 978-1-4697-9514-0 (sc)
ISBN: 978-1-4697-9515-7 (ebk)

Printed in the United States of America

iUniverse rev. date: 03/01/2012

This Book is dedicated to

My first love and best friend

Gail

and a very special thank you to my kindest and dearest of friends

Ingrid

and thank you also to a very warm kind soul the daughter of Gail

Summer

And to those who do not understand gender dysphoria or a person like myself who has a crossed gender, and I have hurt you, scared you away, and made you angry, I have cried a billion tears trying to find the answer for you and myself, and will cry a billion tears still if not more, As an offer to you as payment back to let you know, how much it hurts me and I am in pain, knowing that I have hurt you more than myself

Sincerely
Cynthia Marie

A real story about the struggle for life and identity who as a child who realizes he//she is not the correct gender and knowing everyone around this child, does not want "it" to have the identity, "it" knows belongs to "it" the life long struggle to have "it", keep "it" lock "it" up safe, and to grow into an empathetic being, knowing that a soul has pain it may carry a long way with "it" after even "it's" time here. and feeling it from others, hurts more than your own, if you were the cause, being one they chose, and not the one you were meant to be, and grow in a world you do not belong in, Somewhere in birth you were made as special, I remember my birth, my short time in my womb, safe! a feeling of floating in a warm sea of twinkling stars, in the warm heart of the heavens, and the soft beautiful music surrounds every part of being here, the musical symphonies played on the golden and wooden handmade instruments of the heavens, music from the angels own voices surround and comfort, a tiny new little soul hanging in balance by a small thread of gold. Waiting to fall into the chaos of the cold earth below, in search again, for that warm safe feeling that will only come one time in a moment, after a long life of endless emotional violence, storms calm and winds comfort in a gentle breeze. Sail's in a chance to breathe again, look, feel, and, embrace, and awaken to feel safe and warm, again, a gentle touch, gentle as a kiss to push forward, "love", this time, herself!

Then it went dark, and then onto a big bright opening I was standing in front of a large window looking out! Seeing two small children playing in snow, I asked my mother who they were, she said! Your sisters!, don't you recognize your own sisters? all my memories flooded me, I had awaken, for the first time, I had become aware of myself, and my memories of living in Worlds End, in Hingham Massachusetts. Where Out my back door I could walk across a dirt road and walk out into one of the most beautiful of the new England Parks, A small group of tiny islands nestled off Hingham Harbor, where my life begins and from then on as I choose to be who I am, the dislikes, the hate, the beatings, the humiliation, the constant bullying, blackouts, keeping it to myself, or the boys I had to associate or play with every day would look at each other for weakness and then you became a target for bullying and beatings, I sensed very early at that time there was a lot of feeling wrong about it, as if I had learned it was wrong before I knew it was, something I would have been taught by someone at an earlier age two to three years old, someone like my parents! They knew? I always speculated in my life if they did, but later in life would find out that in fact they did. And would get to the point of even using force to mold me into their son, I was the son they both wanted, especially my mother, she wanted me badly as she would always repeat that, she had two girls first then me, in my family having the son first is a great thing, an honor, so they had to wait hoping the third was the son they awaited for was me.

And here I was, not their son but there daughter but as a tiny infant in my mother's arms, all she saw was a little boy, and she wanted to keep that moment forever, I was taken from her at birth for a few hours they said I was a blue baby, when they gave me back she was told to treat me very gently, I will always be very fragile, but he did not say why. They bought me the all best of toys, I admit! Being a boy, you really got some cool stuff. I remember at three years old opening a Christmas present and pulling out a complete set of Yellow Tonka trucks, everything a boy would want and everything you would need on any construction site as a grown up to build a city, I do remember playing with them in the dirt but later they would be all broken, my mom said I busted them all, but I don't remember doing it and these where tough old Tonka trucks made in the early 1950's. how could they get broken by such a small boy like myself, later I would find out what may have happened to them, but

2

that's when I went into Hingham High much later in life, and the surprise I got when I talked to an Old neighborhood kid I had remembered from Worlds End. It was a shocking surprise and a revelation to an answer I was seeking for so long, it helped me start to understand how far back all this confusion about my gender went. And also my mother said I had a doll I loved the most, named baby blue, I carried it everywhere I went, When I was six years old, just for old times, bought me another, I remembered it, My dad was good in the beginning we had a good relationship, He gave me his old Junk cars to play in, I wish I had one of those nice old antique cars now, In the driveway for rides on Sunday and a parade, he brought me to his work a couple times on a Saturday, One Friday I had tied my toy car to his bumper and hoped to get up early and have him tow me behind his car to work, but I over slept, he was laughing so hard when he found my little car tied to his bumper that morning, that's when I told him my plans, so he told me he would bring me in his car instead, I remember playing in those old cars I was so small I had to stand on the seat to reach the steering wheel, And picking blueberries in the woods with my sisters, also running to the bus stop and looking behind me as my mother followed behind with a hair brush, to keep me moving along, and getting to the bus stop where I would see groups of older boys 6-7 years old looking at me and laughing, girls huddled together and just watching, I would feel like I was leaving my body, I don't ever remember getting on any bus, For a short time at the age of three to four years of age I stayed with an aunt in Medford MA, My mothers, mothers sister, my mother came to me and asked me, she said, your aunt cannot have any babies and wants to know if you would like to stay with her, maybe they will adopt you, she is so sad! She wants to have a child so bad will you go and be with her? And see if you would like to stay? I said yes! right away. I wanted to help, and I loved it there, my aunt was so nice to me, and one thing I remember and loved the most was bedtime, she put me in a little nightgown she said do you mind wearing that? It is just like what your mommy wore to bed when she was a little girl, and I said sure it's fine.

I did not mind, I had no idea but I liked it and slept so good after she tucked me in She always kissed my forehead, only, my uncle was mean, he complained I was there, I heard him say why is he here? Why we are taking care of and feeding there kid? And would tease me when I ate

some ice cream, he would say! That was mine, you ate the ice cream I
wanted, my aunt would tell him to leave me alone, but he never would,
I broke down and cried one day after listening to another fight about
me, and another day of his mean teasing, and went back home, not that
I really wanted to, I know how much it hurt my aunt, I cried as much or
maybe more than her when I left, I felt I abandoned her and left her
alone with a mean man in the house and no baby, and I brought her so
much joy, but my uncle was just to mean, and a few years later my aunt
died of a heart attack, I thought I broke it, It was the first funeral I
would go to in my life, I cry so much at funerals now, I always wondered
later what that was about, I was about three maybe four years old, did
she or my parents know something and hoped moving me out of the
neighborhood was a good thing to do? And why me I thought, I was the
son she always wanted, why give me away, so young,? And this aunt
was the right place to send me? And dressing me as a girl at bed time, I
loved it! I still remember that, It is such a fond memory and I always
think of it when I remember her, We always went back to visit on
holidays but I was shy to talk to her I felt I really hurt her leaving her
without a baby, At the age of five we moved from Hingham to Hull Ma,
My dad had to work more and I saw little of him, I may have spent as
many days with him as I can count on one hand, My life in Hull was
going to be a lonely trial in fire, My first day in kindergarten as I waited
for everyone to come to class I was alone about half an hour, I came
with my sisters on their bus, they went in earlier, the first into the
classroom after me was a girl, she introduced herself to me, her name
Mary Lou, she showed me how to trace the dots on my paper at my
desk, when connected spelled your name, she said I love your name,
will you be my friend? You can come to my house and play, and while
she was connecting the dots I got my first feeling of a warm glow as if
she had an aura around her and I sensed her good will. A feeling making
me slightly paralyzed with a warm numbness and a feeling of floating,
it was a very nice, warm feeling, It is a feeling I still get around certain
people, empathetic people, I feel them, I feel there aura coming off
them, as if it were a defense mechanism or sixth sense, something I
developed to feel safe around certain people, and Mary Lou and I
became friends for about one year, We played at her house, she had
everything a play house needed, stoves, counters, sinks, cabinets, a
table to sit and have tea, I had so much fun playing with my friend Mary

Lou and all her nice toys and dolls, Till one day her mother answered the door and said you shouldn't be here playing with a girl and girl toys all the time, you need to play with boys, and boy toys, and sent her little son out to play, a small boy still in diapers, I wanted to play but not with him, I wanted my friend Mary Lou, And Mary and I just looked at each other through the window, after several times I went to play with Mary and was giving her brother instead, I gave up, my friend was taking away by a mother who didn't want a boy playing like a girl. So I just stopped seeing her, how this would so affect me later in life as a lifetime of fear to ever talk to a girl again, The home we moved into in Hull, Ma, was a large Victorian on Nantasket Ave this house had issues, issues with paranormal activities, strange things happened, door knobs turned and twisted and when you opened the door no one was there, People walked up and down the stairs but no one was seen, A small clay tile on the fire place mantle with Jesus impressed on it, It would be facing the wall when we came down in the morning sometimes we found it face down on the brick floor of the fireplace, it never broke, it's as if someone gently put it there, my mother soon put it in a draw, I don't know where it is now, I remember our first night in Hull sitting in a large dark room and a birthday cake was the only light in the room. We had moved in early by one day and no electricity was turned on yet, and because my parents were so busy moving we had all 3 birthdays in one, my two older sisters and I all blew out the candles, and it just went dark, I had my own small room upstairs my two sisters shared another larger room, and my mom and dad and another sister soon to arrive sister number three. In a small room at the end of the hall, One night I woke up freezing cold and had to pee real bad, about 3-4 in the morning, as I opened my eyes I see two tiny little feet in front of my face, tiny little toes and I could see all the little wrinkles in them, and I could even see the tiny toe nails and a blue dress hung low and draped the arches of her feet with a lace trim, As I slowly looked up I saw two small hands hung by her sides. all the little wrinkles in the knuckles of each little finger and tiny small finger nails, all where as clear as day, As I slowly looked up at her I saw a lace trim wrapped around the waste and it matched the very bottom of her dress, As I look further up I see three little blue buttons on the front of her blue dress. And a lace breast area of the dress And a round collar, folded down at the top, no lace trim, on it, at the shoulders there is strawberry blonde hair sweeping across, a tiny little

5

closed mouth just the two red lips closed in a slight smile, and a tiny nose, but! No eyes! where her eyes should be, where just a shadow of them, and though I did not see her eyes, I could tell she was staring right into mine, like she knew she had woken me up, she floated about a foot away from my face, I could have reached right out and touched her, she was surrounded by a bluish aura that lit her up a little, I closed my eyes several times and blinked but she just stayed right there, she would not go away, I thought I was just dreaming this, but she was so real, just like looking at another person clear as day, I got so scared I just kept my eyes closed and eventually went to sleep, peeing was no longer important, I was so scared to open my eyes in the morning and still see her, It was the first time in my life I felt absolute fear as scary as it gets, I would see her many times after that, if I woke up in the night, a lot of times she was at the bottom of my bed just floating there watching me sleep. when she was further away I could see her eyes, and her collar turned up exposing the lace underneath, small tiny little piercing blue eyes just staring at me, she was about the size of a 2 or 3 year old girl but her face looked older like a woman's face, not a young girl, I never told anyone I always thought I was seeing things, it's a dream or something, about a year later I switched rooms, My oldest sister wanted her own room, there where now three girls in one room and another sister on the way to make it four, and me right in the middle, of four sisters what an awful place to be tested, I got a very large room for myself and never saw the little girl any more, And later in my twenties when I was with some of my sisters talking about the old house, my older sister mentioned a little girl, that floated over her watching her sleep at night and she would see her running around playing in the room and would hide in the closet before the sun came up, the skin crawled right off me, she saw her too? She really was there! I tell you the saying the skin crawls off your body is very accurate, the goose bumps I got where so big and tingled so much, I thought all my skin just wiggled right off me, To this day I wake up at night wondering if I will ever see her again but never have, but I do check, I was very happy to move out of that house. I never in my life want to see or hear any of the things I saw heard and felt in that old house. and would have two other encounters later with spiritual beings, not the little girl, I could write a book alone just on the unnatural activities that went on in that house for the years we lived there, scaring everyone, Even my own dad was scared, There where nights we would all get woken up and stand in the upstairs as a group in the hallway, listening to furniture up in the attic moving across the floors along with footsteps, when you opened the door going up to the attic the cold breeze that would come down on would make you want to shut it right away, my dad would not even walk up those attic stares to see what was up there, I learned very early in life that when you die, you go somewhere, there is no end, there is a god, these experiences made me religious at a young age and made me aware that I must be here for some reason, I have no idea what and why and why I am who I am, but I know there is a reason, and I know that god is testing me for some purpose, and I have a soul to protect, A female soul, a woman's soul, but also the guilt that I am doing something wrong, why was I like this and where do I go from here, and now at about the age of six, first grade had begun, I was so scared and shy, the teacher was very mean and strict, And I had learned now that there where rules, for boys and rules for girls, we lined up boy girl boy girl or girls one side of the room boys on the other, I would look at the girls and feel so out of place, I felt like I should be over there with them, That I was a boy because that's what my parents wanted me to be, I would feel mesmerized looking at the girls in there pretty dresses and happy smiles, and feel an out of body feeling all of a sudden I would be in the nurses office like I lost track of time, like a blackout, and I would get sent home, My first crush would happen, Out at recess in the school yard, in first grade, I kept more to myself and played with no one, I brought a tennis ball to school and bounced it off the dug outs, I was not sure who to play with, and one day a girl crippled with polio came walking over to me, she had braces on both legs and used crutches to walk, she asked me to help her put one of her straps back together, it had come loose, so I helped her buckle it up and she just smiled at me, I really thought she could have done it herself but, she was looking for a friend, I fell so in love right there, I hoped she would come back again every day to ask me again to buckle her braces, but never did, and I was so shy I couldn't walk up to her, she stayed by a tree and played under it every day, As with any other girl I would meet I would daydream we would be friends, but I always saw myself as a girl playing with them, Not a boy, I wanted to dress like them and play with them as a girl not a boy, And it was very confusing to me that I thought like that, It made me keep to myself I would just get my feelings hurt or there's and other kids may not like me, and just laugh at me, and their mothers would take them away from me, like my friend Mary Lou, that hurt me when that happened, I got so scared to make friends again, And I always fell for those type of girls after that, Ones that had to wear glasses or had other problems with their health, I wanted to care for them, And be there mommy, My time in first grade was such a failure, they almost kept me back, they said I was not ready for school, but it was, I was always just to scared and shy, I knew who I was and how I felt, and I knew for some strange reason that what I was feeling was wrong, a family lived a few houses away they just moved in, there where twins a boy and a girl, but there sexes where crossed, she acted like a boy and he acted like a girl, he always got beat up but she came out and beat up whoever hurt her brother, I saw what kids did to boys that wanted to be a girl, and I saw him get teased daily, but never the sister, no one dared bother her, they got a beaten, But 2nd grade was so different, the teacher I had treated me like I was special, out of all the boys and girls in my class and grade I was the tiniest, My parents did not think I was going to grow, doctors where concerned about how petite I was, she would let me sit on her lap and gave me lots of attention, I was so in love with this teacher I just wanted to please her every day, I could not wait till school started, Every morning I got up and ran to the bus stop, And it would be the only good year I would ever have in school again. I have always felt that the bond I had and will always have with all the woman in my life came from her, Mr.'s. Epstein, and the need to be with them as a friend and a lover and the want to be nurtured was installed in me that time in my life, by that woman in that moment, she nurtured me away from my home where no one else ever had reached me, I would say she may almost be my first love or real hard crush I had, Only it was just me in love there was no relationship the age difference is 20-25 years apart, but was I in love, and to this day I still have wonderful feelings for her, I would love to see her, I don't know if she would still be alive, But later I had the same teacher that I had in first grade in third, she acted like she would regret having me back in her class, and I flunked everything, I had become withdrawn and could not focus on school again at all, I started to become more aware of the boy girl differences mostly in clothes, bathrooms, gym class, and manners, and was depressed at a very young age, I still had no idea about sexes. And why we are like this as people, why are some boys and why are some girls, and who makes that decision, my parents? And my mom saw how depressed I was, and would lift me up and hug me and say, please tell me what's bothering you, you're my little boy that I waited so long for tell me anything, anything at all you're the son I wanted so bad, but inside I wanted to tell her, I don't want to be your son I want to be your daughter, but I never could, she never really gave me that chance! And sometimes I think she said that because she did know! she was afraid I would tell her I wanted to be her daughter, she should have just said I already know, I want to help you, I was more afraid of hurting her feelings than my own, but I had started to cross dress, I had no idea what that meant then but I knew if I dressed as a girl I had to hide somewhere, and the big house made that easy and there were plenty of girls clothes everywhere. With four sisters, there were dresses all over the house, In my room alone or up in the attic, in the basement, in the bathroom, I would get to dress up, but I knew I had to hide when I did, and the times I dressed up where short, I never did when everyone was home, And walking about the house, and there would be months sometimes in between these little adventures of mine, but when I put a dress on it felt right, I was me, I was who and what I wanted to be, and I could not tell anyone, I was so afraid of being caught I remember the first time, I was going through boxes in the attic, a scary place to be any way, some neighbors from the old neighborhood in worlds end moved and we stored some of their belongings and I found a box full of dresses, 'there was a full length mirror on the wall, I ran and got some of my mom's red lipstick and powder blush and dressed up quick it was my real first time to do this, I don't know why I wanted to so badly but when I saw all those beautiful dresses I had to try them on, it was over fast I did not want to get caught, but that little glimpse I saw of myself that first time, was the first time I looked at myself and felt relaxed, a feeling of comfort and warmth Is a good way to describe it when you recognize yourself for the first time, It's a feeling of looking at a friendly face after being all alone for months I kept that image in my mind like a treasure in a little box, A little secret friend, where I would go in escape in dreams away from places I did not want to be. And I would turn into a girl. and get to be her in my little safe happy place, My child hood was pretty normal with playing in the old neighborhood, it was fun, a good deal of my child hood was ok, I did have a lot of fun playing out on Allenton Hill Hull Ma, we all made buggies like they did on the little rascals television show, and rode them down the hills while someone would stay at the bottom to yell out all clear, no cars where coming, In the winter we used sleds, and the games of hide and seek and war games with toy guns, all the kids joined in to play, boy and girls, we all played together back then, always plenty of kids to play with in large groups. and endless days of summers swimming at the beach, north eastern storms washed lobsters ashore and we had a lot of cook outs, and relatives would fill the house with all the parties we had, The fifties and early sixties where a great time I was going to grow up in the hippie generation, The Beatles have been on the Ed Sullivan show and kids where changing their old hair styles, now it was time a boy could have longer hair but not me my parents would make me cut my hair, like a ritual, my mom saw one hair coming over my ears and I got put into a chair, To get it all chopped off, I hated it, I wanted long hair and I started to rebel, my dad would slap me if I didn't get in and sit still, While my mom pushed those electric clippers through my hair, he would stand there and make sure I did not move a muscle. If I cried I got teased, what's the matter want to be a little girl? As my sisters would point at me and giggle, and laugh and tease me, even my mother, while my hair was being ripped away from my head, saying oh good you don't look like a little girl anymore, with each haircut, and I could not say anything, never, not a whisper, just a little voice inside crying for help, But it was just a lonely voice inside, my little friend in her box trying to scream out but no one could hear her, I was too scared to tell anyone, That little picture I had of myself in my mind the first time I got dressed in the attic I put in a little box and became a safe place to go when pain came, soon the box got bigger and more beautiful inside and the girl inside grew along with me, as I grew she did also, but she became a woman and I did not, I had just started 4th grade and was not in school long, about a month and then they took me out of school they said I was not ready, and said my hearing was very bad, and also I had to have my tonsils out, so my parents took me out of school that year, I had my tonsils out and, they put tubes inside my ear canals to open them up. Hoping I would hear better, it worked for about a month then I could not hear good again, this time it was real, They scarred my ear drums putting those tubes in and really made me deaf, I wasn't deaf before, I was just so sad and depressed and I had just faded out. I could not speak much or hear much, I just felt lost inside of daydreams hoping someday I will get to be a girl, I hoped somehow somewhere there was an answer, I even hoped aliens in spaceships would come down from the skies and find me, Read my mind and fix me, then drop me back on the planet as a girl, but how was I to explain that, And the worst was still to come, each year in school was worse than the last, As I learned more about the physical difference, between boys and girls, but still not sexual yet, I had not made the female male connection, All I knew was I had something attached to me they didn't, a penis! And why that made a difference I did not know then, but I had one, and I did not want to have it. I hoped it was going to fall off like a loose tooth or disappear back up inside me; this thing attached to me was a problem. Why did this little thing attached to me offer such great reward as a boy, it was a lock, I watched a cartoon one day and the characters where helping out a friend with a bad tooth, they tied a string around the tooth and then a door knob and slammed the door shut, And out popped the tooth, what an idea, could I do that? Too this part I don't want on me? I tried it, I put a string on a door knob and then tied it around my extra part in hopes that I could get rid of it but when I tightened the string up on myself the pain was so bad, I doubled over and fell, ooooo that hurt and it took more than a few minutes to get that string off too, I gave up that idea, what a painful experience that was both mental and physical, I still had to deal with this part of me I didn't want, I was about eight years old when I did that, I still feel that when I remember it, I was living with my grandmother the year before I returned to school, she took me home from the hospital and I stayed that whole year into the next fall, but I had to leave and go back and try the fourth grade again, I loved staying with my grandmother she was very kind and went out to shop a lot, so I had time to myself a lot, and my grandfather just stayed downstairs, My grandmother had a nice table and mirror in her room All filled with makeup, lipsticks, powder's, and brushes, there where small slips to wear and hats, I wonder if she ever knew I was playing with her stuff, I bet she did, she was meticulous and neat, but she never said anything and I cleaned up as best as I could, But she was one to notice anything out of place, I loved lipstick the most as a child, the change it made in my looks was so comforting, I loved it! I did not look like me anymore I was her, just with that, I learned some things watching her and then when she left I tried to imitate what she did, and hid a few things for myself, when I was going home I had a little stash of make up in my clothes mostly lipsticks, and when my grandmother picked up my clothes they all fell on the floor, and my mom was standing right there, they just looked at each other, my grandmother said what were you doing with those?, I told her I was bringing them home for my mommy, and she just smiled at me And said I have been looking all over for that stuff, so that's where it is, To this day the smell of finishing powder reminds me of her, and she taught me how to cook and eat eggs, boiled, hard and soft, poached, and fried, and all good vegetables, like broccoli and asparagus's, Brussels sprouts, cauliflower, I never had these and with real butter, my mom just made the same old mixed vegetable or just peas and carrots, whatever my sisters would like, and there were four of them so they won out, and I never got many vegetables as a child, I hate peas and carrots still, But that time went fast and soon had to return to hull, into the fourth grade again, and I had the meanest teacher in the school for home room, He was so cruel that if one kid in class spoke out wrong, or disrupted the class at all, we were all punished, He would take us out at recess and make us stand at attention in the coldest windiest place he could find. If one kid wiped there runny nose, or cried, or moved one muscle, we would be back out there again and again and again, for weeks sometimes nonstop, that's all I remember about that year, was the cruelty of this teacher He watched us like hawks as he walked up and down between the aisles of desks always jingling the change in his pocket it looked like he was rolling dice in his pant pockets, and as soon as one kid did something wrong all us would get punished, to this day I can't figure out why the other teachers and the principal allowed this type of cruelty to go on like it was nothing, but a lot of the teachers where bad, my mother had many fights with them with my sisters ahead of me and when they got me in there class and remembered my mother, some acted out revenge, I saw him again when I was seventeen working part time, in a small store, as a clerk in Hingham he was a tiny little man about 4 and a half feet tall and as homely as a little monkey, I just stared at him, I could not help it, I knew it was him, his name was on his shirt tag, He looked frightened and he trembled when I stared at him, as if he knew he was recognized by a former student, and I saw what a puny weak little man he really was. He must have felt good torturing all of us, to get back for what he went through with some mean old wife at home, or all the bullying he took as a child, all the kids in school called him the monkey man, and now I saw why? And! The worst was still to come. Even by 5th grade I had no idea about" sex" still, the fact men and woman connected to each other, I was so scared, I was afraid to move, or talk, carry my books the wrong way, walk wrong, use my hands wrong, I had become so paranoid especially with my body language, I thought out every move I made and it takes a lot of your energy and learning process away, Fifth grade was when I reached a point suicide became an option, depression was making its way in and becoming a feeling stronger than the others I had, and winning, There were a few kids in town that we lost from suicide they through with it, for why I don't know, One kid called a priest and told him he was going to hang himself, when the priest got there it was too late, But, I learned of an option, A way out, And one day pushed too far to a point I just broke down. I sat and cried at a lunch table and told three teachers I can't take it anymore I want to die, they just stared with blank faces, One said toughen up it's part of life, just another day to get through, you can do it! if I had a gun in my pocket I would have taken it out and blew my brains out, but all they would have done is call the janitor to clean up before calling my mother or the police, I find now when someone commits suicide a piece of me goes with them, even strangers, I feel a loss myself, and I know I felt there pain, they left and gave up trying, it takes a lot of pain and loneliness to give up and leave, I wish I could have just told someone, anyone, But the teachers trying to break through where not kind in there manner, but aggressive and used humiliation and punishment for not answering there questions, I always wondered why they kept me back in the fourth grade, Why did they all of a sudden pull me out of school, I was very athletic, It all seemed ok to me at the start and I had a nice teacher! and I had met that week, a girl, that would later be my most intimate of friends, and remains to this day Right in the hall I will never forget, I was the only kid in my grade that climbed the rope all the way to the top and touched the ceiling and could keep doing it while kids who bullied me cried or where too scared to even try, some got about ten feet up, They were only tough in numbers, and I was fast, I had very fast reflexes, they had a test, you had a ruler dropped between your fingers and you had to pinch it quick or it hit the floor, I beat everyone by inches, ninety seven percent of the entire grade dropped it, a science teacher did the experiment, he was shocked I did so well and said I was lucky and had me do it again, only to be better, at the speed of my reflexes, and fourth grades first few weeks of my first attempt at it I did not think were too bad, And I never would have had to deal with that monster of a teacher in home room I had when I returned after my throat and ear surgery Which was strange how it all happened my sister was complaining of a sore throat, not me, the doctor examined her found nothing and said to me let's see how you look and said, you are the one with the bad throat and winked at my parents, I just came to watch not get examined, this was not my appointment, so I thought, next thing I know I am taken out of school and sent to the hospital, It didn't seem right, seemed planned, seemed like taking my sister in was a decoy, it was me they wanted, and they said I would hear again real good but they made me worse they scarred my ear drums and I have lost 50 percent of my hearing now, and will lose more in the work I do as an adult, And I as am entering the 6th grade, they change the school hours and split it into two shifts, I was put on second so I went to the bus at noon time, the day before school starts a kid from the neighborhood calls, I knew and played with at times was a kid known to police by the age of ten by twelve years old had a record as long as his arm, a real Dennis to menace type kid, he calls me, and said he was on 2n'd shift for the double sessions with me. And said come on over and let's talk there is another kid here also, let's all meet up, so we all know who we are with at the bus stop, so I said sure, be right over, I knock at the door and my friend is laughing in hysterics on the floor just rolling, I say what's so funny? He said look in the television room quick, so I walk in, first I see the television on, then I look to my left and there is this boy on a couch with his pants down around his knees, masturbating, I was shocked! I had no idea what that was and why he was doing that, I turned and walk out real quick embarrassed and confused all in one, And now my other friend while still laughing tells me in an instance, all and everything there was to know about sex and why the boy, girl thing! And what it was all about, I was horrified! I felt for the first time in my life I would be forever trapped! In an identity and body I did not belong in, the reality cut through me like a cold dull knife, I don't think I spoke a word for a month, Making the beginning of the sixth grade hell, and because of double sessions I was now with kids from the other side of town, kids I never saw in my life, strangers. 90 percent of the school where all new faces, and in that town kids broke off into little street gangs every little area was a territory for groups of boys and if you mistakenly walked into a group of them alone in their neighborhood and they caught you, you got a beating, I have been beat down to the ground kicked punched beaten with shoes, have had kids break sticks over my back, and not fairly, a group of four to five held you and beat you while the rest watched, and helped push you back down when you tried to get up, The worst was in the village at the old fort warren at the top of the cemetery, there where manholes in the floor where water once flowed through the fort for plumbing and some tunnels to hide ammo, If you went there at the wrong time of the day near night time, and walked by a couple manholes kids would pop up out of them and you would be surrounded. If you didn't get away you got the beaten of your life, and by much older kids. My brother got a real bad beaten once up there, but me I saw them coming up out of the manholes and one got stuck, And I ran before they got out, and was chased at high speed down a cemetery hill jumping and dodging tomb stones and was chased another ½ mile before, who was ever chasing me stopped, boy can you run fast when you are scared, and Now I had to go to school with all the kids that where not of my neighborhood I was alone and scared of what I just saw happen with those boys masturbating, it was nothing to them, and a few times when I went over there, to meet up for school, there were more of them, lots of them practicing and all of at once all of them playing with it, experimenting, one brought his sister for everyone to practice on, and some practiced on each other, I stopped going there it had a very scary, and evil feel to it, and I feel I may have eventually been forced to do something I did not want to do, boys and their penis's and the things they do with them, when they are learning, I was so scared what the hell had happened, I looked like I must have been somewhere else on some other planet, I told my friend rick what was going on over there, he did not know too much either, and I hung with him much more after that, he was always the friend I could talk to, we should have been brothers if I was really a boy, he was always sad he lost his brother to a diseases, he never told me the exact illness, but he grieved a lot as a child for his brother, Nicky, and he was called Ricky, He to this day is still my most trusted male friend and one I can talk to about intimate things in my life about, but he was a grade ahead of me I was not with him in school, I was all alone I knew very few people, I was lost, and I was getting the bullying of my life By students even teachers who would say when you asked for help, It's just a part of life toughen up learn to fight back. my first day sixth grade in math class all there was were red pens in home room, we were all out of pencils, we did a short exam to see what we remembered, and I had every answer right, except the teacher through a fit I dare use a pen in math class, she said what are you so smart you don't need an eraser? You don't make mistakes? and you used "red" that's my color for correcting papers, only I use that color, I told her why I used the pen but she did not care she took my pen and gave me a big "F" on my paper picked it up and showed it to the class as an example, to let everyone know, I flunked her class that year, I was so scared to move as things just got worse like I was frozen in time, If these kids saw signs of being girly the results would be a beating after school or in the hall or restrooms, mostly the boys bathrooms were a bad place to be, I could not pee standing at the urinals I needed to sit, and if you do that and peed in the boys room, and they discovered you, it got around fast, it is amazing at how young an age boys look for the girly boy, so they can hurt him, I froze in fear every time I entered a room with kids in it, I had become so withdrawn and so quiet and unresponsive. One teacher told me to get up and recite the alphabet, just to see if I knew it, how humiliating, everyone was watching and looking at me saying come on you can do it, cheering me on, I got up and walked out of the class then out the side door of the school and went home, they gave me detention but I would not go to it, I got out some side door somewhere, a lot of truancy soon started, I missed so much school I had to go to summer school but I, skipped most of that, they just passed me along to the 7th grade just to get rid of me, and that summer just before 7th grade, I was sitting on a rowboat in a neighbors backyard looking out over hull bay, And wondering what all this was about, When the next thing I know is I am down on the ground in a headlock And my head was being squeezed so hard the pain was like an electric shock next thing I know I wiggled out and stood toe to toe for at least a ten minute all out punching kicking fist fight with a neighborhood kid I had seen around but did not know, we just punched each other till we got tired and he said whoa now, you're not the little wimpy kid I heard you where, you fight pretty good, my name is Tony, lets hang out, what do you want to go do? and from then on in I had a friend I would know the rest of my life, almost, he does not accept me now, he always made remarks about gays and homos, he hated them, thought they should all be murdered, We raked leaves and shoveled walks and always found work to make a little money to hang out and play pinball at the corner store, we had no video games pinball was modern, I have to say he put a you have to work hard to get money ethic in me, that I always had after that, Tony and another neighborhood kid Rick I met at seven years of age, And later a good friend Steve, a couple years older than us, joined in, these would be my three main child hood friends, who I hung out with, A little pack, and from there I met other kids in the town I never would have gotten to know ever, and being in this group gave me a place, I could walk more freely about the town without the risk of getting a beaten and I also started down a bad path, Some of these kids where the ones breaking in houses, stealing cars, in and out of juvenile hall, To hang out with them meant doing things I never thought I would be doing, Not my three friends as much as who we started to mix with, I thought of it as my new beginning into becoming a "boy",a "man", even a chance that I would grow away from these feelings and would be normal, the feelings of being a girl would disappear now, I had a way of growing to try and get it out of my head, I would do everything a boy would do and become a man in life and keep the feelings I had, pushed down, way inside so they would hopefully disappear, for a long time I kept my feelings inside, like I put a heavy weight on those dreams and let it drop way down into my brain and kept them there. At least that's what I thought, but as soon as I was inactive, And had time to wander off in a dream, or daydream she came back, And I would resist it and put her away again, in that little box, and I would see her banging on the sides of the box and jumping up and down, let me out, let me out, I am you, let me out, I had to stop thinking like that if I wanted friends and I wanted to make something of my life, the kids I hung with hated anyone who would be different, gays, especially, and any boy that dresses like a girl or acted like one was to get a beaten, Some talked of killing, they would be doing the world a favor, And I had to sit there and listen to this talk, it frightened me, They were serious about doing harm to people that thought like me! I felt like a woman with a group of men, being told they were going to rape me, and kill me, while I sat there and listened to them talk, about their plans And I took that seriously And would spend another 20 years as a man trying to be one, and be the best man I could be, though 7th and eighth grade where my lost years in school I skipped repeatedly I was hardly there, I did very little cross dressing maybe every other month once or twice for only a few moments just minutes, I never had the privacy and time alone with such a house full of kids there were seven of us now. I had two younger brothers, and by the beginning of ninth grade. I had been sought after by the truant officer. He saw me playing at the beach and I ran, After that he had my name on top of the list, and my mother said "go get him", she did not help me and she knew how badly I was treated in school, she blamed me, and I was eventually brought to court. I was told by a judge not to miss one more day without a real good reason, or I am going into a juvenile facility till I turned eighteen, I was just fifteen, then my life takes a strange turn, as I am walking to school one morning in late November, I had no coat on just a sweater, I could no longer bear the thought of wearing the clothes my parents bought me, it looked like I stepped out of a forties television show, I had just confronted my father the day before when I told him I don't want to wear what he wears, He always wore those Dickie work pants, and that's what they bought me, I hated them, they are so uncomfortable, I wanted jeans and shirts like the kids in school had. He went nuts, he said those jeans those tight jeans the kids were wearing? Showing everything they got, what are you? Some type of queer! Some queer little fag wanting to show your stuff you want to show your stuff to men don't you? Then he beat the shit out of me, real bad, He said no son of mine is ever going to look like a fucking queer or ever be one, I said no! I just want to look like everyone else and fit in, but he would not even listen, He had a gleam in his eyes they looked like shiny glass eyes, as if he replaced them with marbles, I see that in people that hate, and I have seen it in people that use to know me and see me now, I know they are the ones to watch out for, He kicked me and punched me all over my room till he got to tired and left, that was the most painful, hurtful beating I ever got, more emotionally than anything else, The physical pain I barely felt at all, but my own father accusing me of being gay then beating me was horrible, I am not gay, He often beat me whenever I did something to get my mother mad, and it wouldn't take much, just someday I would look at her wrong, and sometimes I felt so black mailed in a way, she would say do this or when dad gets home I will see to it that you get a beaten you will never forget, when dad came home everyone else would be down stairs jumping up and down all excited daddy is home but not me, ` I was upstairs shaking and trembling, waiting for those heavy footsteps coming slowly up the stairs as I waited for the beating my mother told my dad to go give me, no jeans for me. Until I saved my own money, And I would not wear the coat they bought me to school I would rather freeze to death, Every time I did I got made fun of. Or got a beaten from someone, so on this long cold walk to school a man standing on a porch, He says don't you have a coat young man, Aren't you cold, it's freezing out! I look up and see this large bald man with a grin on his face, like the chestashere cat. And I said no! I don't have one, my parents can't afford to buy me one, he did not say anything just looked. And I turned and walked off to school, But I knew this man, he was an artist In town who had a reputation for being extremely loony and crazy and was rumored a child molester and a queer, I had remembered him from the other neighborhood kids who would go down to his house and get 7-10 bucks if you let him take pictures of you in a bathing suit and he would paint your portraits, in beach scenes, and inside his house was full of decorations and posters, black lights, everywhere, everything inside the house glowed or sparkled, I went there about a year before with a group of friends who wanted spending money for the weekend you know like beer and pot, and other drugs now available in the early sixties, I had not yet tried these things but soon would, just like everyone else in that time would. On a walk back from school one day I stop in to talk, and he Is very friendly and welcoming, We talked about who each of us where, we walked out to the beach and collected driftwood, that's how he heated his home, The fire place and the gas stove, He had no central heating and he could not really use his basement much, when we got northeasters the waves broke over the sea wall and flooded his cellar, we thought a few times we were going to float away during some of the storms I was at his house, at the time when they came in, I learned when you burn driftwood you got all types of colors in the flames, from the minerals, He liked it when I visited him I was so quiet and polite, He said for the first time ever he could paint with someone in his house, Did you ever get told your reason for living has a purpose, god has plans, you can never guess which ones, until they become obvious, The meeting with this artist and befriending him was the beginning of a change in both our lives as if it were meant to happen. I would get a ride home from him one day, He had asked me if I wanted one, it was cold and he was going out to shop, so I got home ok, but our family dog was out and somehow he ended up hitting it with his car, He got out to help, The injuries were not bad just some road burn, and he went and met my mom, the two talked, and later he would walk or ride his bike back to our house frequently, And talk to my parents, who later became good friends, we all did, even my mother's brother got to meet him and they became fast friends, my uncle my mother's oldest brother and my grandmother bought paintings to help get him going again. It was all going well but it would get a little crazy, Our artist friend had a drinking problem and the kids who were once making a few bucks posing for photographs, where now hanging there and getting drunk, kids 15 years old some even younger some a little older, and he lost control of it all, he was getting robbed blind, The kids got him so stiffed up he was just about handing it all to them, I was told by a kid there that they were all coming back that night time to beat him seriously and rob him for everything he got, I got some of my friends to help, thank god for the fight on the rowboat that day, a group of my friends confront them and said to leave him alone, Anything happens we tell the police who you are, or we will come and get you ourselves, \So that stopped things from getting to serious, and a lot of these kids hanging around there would soon be kicked out, and away for good, a friend who dated my sister stayed there a lot and helped him recover, and kept those bad kids away for good, My artist friend was safer but now, there were no more kids for photographs, no one, he made no new paintings and was getting himself drunk flat on the floor again and no food, I found him one day after school I had stopped by to check on him he was out cold lying on the floor, I took his keys and wallet, locked the house and went and told my mother, who held onto his wallet till he was recovered, and said just watch him, when he wakes up bring him down all this food. He slept on the floor for two days and I got him to wake up on the third, he was so passed out drunk. But I knew he was alive because he had such a loud snore, when he awoke he just grabbed the food I had in a bowl and just ate it! No spoons! Forks! Nothing! Just grabbed it and ate everything in what looked like a couple bites with his hands, The next day had enough strength to get back up and go out and thank my mother for helping, And now he was in bad need of someone to pose for his paintings He asked me but I had said no I am way 'to shy', then he asked my mother and father if I could, and how he needed someone he can trust and kept calling the house and coming over pleading with them to talk me into helping him, even to the point my sisters where saying go ahead, go help him, even my parents said ok! go help the guy out It's ok we know he is safe and all the rumors about him where all lies, So I did, all of a sudden here I am posing in front of a camera a tiny bikini type bathing suit, a girls bathing suit bottom, the first time I was so flushed with embarrassment, but then decided to look at it that, I was doing it professionally and to help a friend in need, and it went well I helped him for a few years get a restart, we became good friends, and to me he was the father figure in my life that I never had, he had a reputation as a queer artist and a molester of children, all crazy talk, he was the kindest gentlest man I would ever know, He never would ever do things people said about him and write about him later in life, I was upset and wrote to anyone putting information on him out there later after his death, and made sure it is corrected, I want his history to be correct, No one knew him as well as me, and a small hand full of close friends, but I knew him right in the cusp of his change no one else did, there was a complete year the two of us hung out together almost nonstop like I lived with him, He wanted to stop drinking, it was killing him, and he smoked tobacco, But soon realized how bad they were and how they were destroying his life, He went out to the islands and picked wild herbs and plants and made teas and smoked some, then he had found new drugs that kept him in a happier state of mind, He used lsd and Marijuana His paintings now changed and he went into a lot more a landscape and scenic style of painting, Leaving the paintings of male figures alone for a while and started on a path of painting all new works instead He had met a whole new group of friends and people and his status as a new artist started to come through, he met a friend from a group of people I knew and developed a great friendship and would travel to Jamaica very frequently with him, His life from then just took a complete turn around and he is now becoming a sought after artist of late, But he had died too young, the lsd he took raised his blood pressure to high and his aorta had one large crack in it from top to bottom, If he had kept drinking back then, he had less than a year left, He was defecating blood and vomiting it also, he could drink down two gallons of rum in a 24 hour period, till he finally passed out. at least now he got another twenty years or more and is missed by many people, He never knew the struggle I had with my gender, It was something I wanted to talk to him about but he had died, Just a few years from when I was ready for the world As a woman, I wish I could have told him I felt like I owed him that, he was in my life when my father was not, He replaced him, and he was a real good friend when you really needed him, once when walking home from school some kids I was with vandalized a park and got caught, And I did not do anything, but they would not speak up and defend me, So I had to pay 66,00 within six months or go to jail, My parents knew I did not do It, but would not pay the fine, and where getting ready to let me go to jail. They seemed glad they had a way to get rid of me, teach me a lesson or something, but my artist friend was so concerned and knew how bad that would have been for me paid my fine and kept me out of jail, I will never forget that, It would have destroyed me, That was the crucial point in our meeting for me, me not going to prison at a young age, and for something I did not do and was so emotionally abused, I never would have survived the first twenty four hours, and when I ever got out, if I did without committing suicide, I never would have ever spoken to either of my parents again ever in my life, but still in my first year of ninth grade I had become so confused and walking into that first day I just did not look at anyone and hardly spoke, In English class one day I tied the curtain string in a hangman's noose while daydreaming about suicide, my English teacher got in my face, first he asked me a series of questions, like what's a noun? An adjective I said I don't know! I said I don't know to all and everything he asked, he got frustrated and swore if he has anything to do with it, He will keep me back in the ninth grade till I was eighteen and when I am eighteen then he would throw me out of school. And I would never get a diploma, and he kept his word, I passed ok, enough to graduate easily, but he stepped in and stopped it, I had to repeat the ninth grade, because a teacher snapped one day and would not give in to what he said he would do. and that first year in high school no matter what I did I was going to fail, I could have had all A's he still would have kept me back somehow for flunking English, Another assistant principal, I would also never forget was in middle school, I was being dismissed early, My friend Rick and I were going someplace and when I got to school the time was changed to half hour earlier, so I changed the time on the note, my mom got a call and she told them what time she wrote, the assistant principal called me in his office and grabbed me by my neck lifted me up slammed me into his lockers and told me I was never to be trusted and would be a loser for the rest of my life, he said he once trusted me now he never would, I never forgot that, I told my parents, it angered them he grabbed my neck like that but they did not do anything, and my mother said if he called when I was with him to explain, there should have been no problem. I had friends some good close friends in the beginning of high school to get by and keep this feeling that still kept coming back, from revealing itself, all the girls in high school where all getting well developed, and the changes going on with my self where emerging sexually, I started having erections a lot, and found it horrible, I knew it was coming but when it did it was worse than I thought it would be, looking at any woman or girls my age was hard. I knew I did not want a boyfriend, uh, uh I was not at all interested in them, I hung with them I knew what they were like inside and how and what they thought about woman, and their girlfriends, most just used them, it was like I was a secret spy on men for woman for myself, it just really seemed nonproductive, and men really seemed like rats, And untrustworthy in a relationship once they finish, they want to leave, and most do, it's really how they feel. A lot do, I know! I have lived with them, worked with them, hear what they say about woman and there male egos are horrible, I have come not to like them very much, and would never look for any romance with this sort! A lot of them scared me This is my outside nurturing with my male friends That 10 to 15 percent difference I find with others like myself, And how you grow up and who you associate with means something, I had read in some cases male lovers are actually very rough with each other and sex can become very violent, many are football players, and bullies, and that may be why they hate us so much is if we win in the end they too have to come out in the open as well it frightens them, I believe that to be true, and I want no part of it, An erection gives a feeling of power and the feeling to dominate, when chemicals are released in your brain, I want to feel kindness and all the gentleness I can get out of embracing anyone or someone, and I will only get that from a woman, although I admit I am a woman and I have to admit to my crushes, all of them, I have to be truthful in this book or it serves no one, and the ones I have had with males, they have been usually unexpected and surprising but just as good as a crush on a woman, two were doctors, one an ear doctor one was an eye doctor, and they both did the same thing and acted the same way they were both quiet and polite, very polite, They had manners, They were concerned and gentle in there touch and speech, and they both pull down a chart with a blown up picture of the part of the body they are examining, and take out a three foot pointer with the rubber tipped point and touch it to each little part of my ear or eye which ever we are there to day to look at and explain in laymen's terms so I understand everything they tell me, and they seem so happy to do this, to take the time to explain every little detail of what we are looking for and why I am experiencing what I am and what needs to be done and why, They are teaching me out of kindness and I have watched a few draw very skillfully. And the look on their face as they drift into their thoughts to put down on paper what they see, in gentle stokes of a pencil, I got that feeling of floating. I know what it is it's my heart opening a little door to let someone in, and that's when I get that feeling of floating, I feel there aura like I did my with first little friend Mary Lou when she helped me in school that first day in kindergarten connect the dots to my name, I believe Mary may have been the first time in my life a stranger out of nowhere came up to me and was so kind, that it forever installed in me a feeling I would have of a strong wonderful spiritual awakening when that simple kind act or any act of genuine kindness, was giving to me or I feel that person is in their own special thoughts, and she was as she traced out the dots, I just look at her face and it is in a dream, drifting off in some pleasant memory, and I know that if I complete this journey and meet a man with the talent and ability to reach my heart that way, he has a chance, and these men were not handsome or muscular they were weak and shy, But talented and sincere in there manner, and had manners, that is so important, I myself do, I am always treating a lady like I would want to be treated myself if I were one, but I have always been honest, and I know just like the woman in my life I want to love I will always break hearts, I cannot get away from that, and my own is the one that is broken always the most, It just stays broken, it is never going to heal, if not yet! not for a long time, It may take the first moment I am allowed as a woman into the hands of god and I be allowed cry a tear in heaven, My role in any embrace was for reproduction, my religious beliefs are very strong, I believed in god and I protect my soul, no one else but myself will, And I actually came to a point that still in my life, even now, that I spend at least 90 percent of my time asking and praying for the help to get by every day, And without that, there may have been things that I did I would be ashamed of, then or later in life, I did not want anything I did, to follow me into the future, I was always afraid of what was ahead, I had developed so many suicidal thoughts that, making a wrong decision now would come back to haunt me later with guilt, and be a reason I would stay in deep depressed mood to actually want and finally commit the act, I thought of my future a lot, especially where I am going to fit in and I knew I will never be normal, I want to stop thinking there is a girl inside me, Watching x-rated films and pictures of the type I strongly felt the woman's part; it was very sexually arousing, what the hell was going on with me? And why did that happen to me, I could not get aroused anytime at all if I put myself in the man's place, nothing, and not only that I hated how they treated the woman in those movies, but if I thought about being the woman it was overwhelming, It made it difficult to approach girls or woman as I knew the feelings in me may come out in the tender acts of love making. any girl or woman I dated or went out with I felt that I had to tell them how I felt, and that I knew I faced a lot of rejection, but I had to be right up front tell any girl I was going to go out with about these feelings I had deep inside, maybe one day I would find an understanding woman who would share in my sexual life, and understand what I was going through, And would nurture that wonderful part of me that was so lonely. We would be wonderful girlfriends, and lovers, It was so strange as I would be getting older and still the same thoughts I had as a small child of being with girls and wanting to look like them in play, was now in my sexual fantasies, I wanted to play with girls as a girl sexually now, "not with dolls", Finding a girlfriend was going to be a long hard process.

And most likely impossible, and it is so hard for me to understand all this, I am kind sincere and I adore the ground a loved one walks upon, as she comes to embrace me, as if a carpet of precious sacred ground made a path to the both of us, and I believe any woman at a young age if you ever find someone like myself and are truly in love, keep him, and let him go where he needs to go but to make sure that he keeps his promise to keep his physical self-intact, so that you as a couple can raise a family, and you will find ways to make adjustments as you go along, he is going to want feminization of his body, so there is a comfort zone in between the clothing, and the times going out in makeup, and you will have a wonderful husband and very loyal spouse for the rest of your life and your children will all be cared for so well, don't be mistaken that a man has to be tough to be a man or a father or a good spouse, but if so cross gendered like myself he or /she can be held onto forever if there is a strong mutual love, and no one fears out siders are judging you, be brave and really just tell them you love him, and mind their own business, the urges to cross dress are very strong with age. Sometimes I felt like I was her just standing there! it was so intense a feeling of being her, but when I snapped out of it I was still me, in boys clothes, But what was now different! If I got dressed I was very aroused, the material of woman's clothing and the stockings and the silks, all are very sensual. I know now why woman love these things, they are sensual beings, and so am I, The very first time I ever masturbated to see what it was like. I was in a dress, and it was actually the most awkward feeling I ever had, very awkward, I t ran down stairs and almost told my mother what I just did, when I got down stairs I just froze, I thought maybe dad I should tell, I was so shocked and surprised by the emotions that I brought to the surface, it scared me, I also thought I may have done it wrong when it hit me I got scared and stopped, that orgasm the first time takes you off the planet, I had no idea that was coming, I heard it was good but my god, and I thought I hurt myself and could not have babies, I was trembling as I stood there watching my mother sweeping the floor, she just looks at me and said is there something you want you look puzzled, and I was feeling so awkward, I was a girl but I felt like I was doing a boys thing, to myself, I felt like I was out of my body, not a feeling I like, masturbation was to be a very difficult part of this life, not only was it a shameful act as I was taught by my peers, parents and everyone around me, you were weak and a loser if you did that yourself, but it was a reality something boys did, they all do, It's part of their life, things I saw boys do with that thing of theirs in front of me and other boys as I grew up, shocked me, where are these values? The myth that no one masturbates is just that! A myth, It just a big secret or something, I never got that one right, and the pain you go through if you do not release it, is horrible, boys call it blue balls, how appropriate, you cannot walk, your testicle's bang together when you walk and you feel like someone is kicking you with each step, the longer you wait the worse it got, And any ejaculation is painful with each release and contraction, there is no enjoyment to it at all, and I hated it I did not want any part of this, and the temptation to go to the kitchen draw and get out a sharp knife and cut it off was a daily thought, and I did not want erections with a dress on, That looked bad, so I would take care of it" before" I dressed and that made dressing easier again, feeling like a boy once I was dressed as a girl, was not what I wanted at all no erections allowed, just peace of mind, "no sexual thoughts to cloud my mind, and distract me from exploring who I was, I could really fully concentrate on who this girl was that was coming out of me and wanting to take over and get rid of the male side of me. At that age 15 years old looking at myself dressed as a woman, standing there was a real comforting feeling, that I felt right, I was me, And the girl I looked at in the mirror was not going away, I love her, and I wanted everyone else to also, I still had ninth grade to go back too and repeat, I was scared out of my mind, I was now with kids a grade back, you think you can handle a younger group easier but it's not that easy, there were still the older kids all there laughing at you because you got kept back, Lucky for me my birthday was coming, I walk into ninth grade in hull for the last time, my sixteenth birthday, I walked in went to the office and said goodbye, I quit, they tried to talk me out of it, said I needed a note from my parents, I said no I don't need any note, I am sixteen the judge said stay in school till your sixteen, and that's just what I am today sixteen, goodbye you never should have done these things to me, you have these last couple years, and you just sat all these years I was abused openly and bullied by jocks and just plain jerks, I would have stayed, Not one of you has ever cared one bit about me, I walk out and later after that, I spent a lot of time with my friend the artist, going out in his boat, To Boston harbor pier 9, a store called the green dolphin, where he hung paintings for sale, always yelling at the owner for not selling anything fast enough, what arguments those two had, then we would go to china town, and eat at the Chinese Restaurants, And other fine dining establishments, He ate things I never heard of like calf brains once he ordered hundred year old duck egg, not really that old but very old, all green on the outside and darker green in the middle, it was horrible, like eating a piece of a rotten old corpse, Ever try blue cheese? One hundred times stronger, but that's just how this guy was, and I accepted it, he said he was a queer artist and he had a reputation for it, That's why he painted boys in those swim suits, and he always got angry and full of anxiety when he would yell that out, it was for the gay community, he said, but it was also an avenue to sell, It was not so true he was such a gay artist, He may have had some gay lovers in his life, I never met any of them, or if I did he did not mention it, he did have some gentleman friends over often, he told my mother he bought the house he lives in because a woman he loved and wanted to marry parked in the lot near the home overlooking Boston Light House, but she withdrew her accepting to his proposal and broke his heart, he never loved another like her again and moved there to remember her, the paintings of male figures is, was what he was good at the time with, but that was to change when one day I go over and he says look what I just bought, pot! Ever try it? I had a couple times earlier but only a couple times, once with my friend Tony we camped on bakers hill when we were kids once ran into a couple a boy and a girl just hanging out said want to smoke with us, and I thought he was smoking tobacco I didn't realize I was smoking pot till it hit me, wow those first few times are awesome, I was young and finding it was risky. Everyone knew everyone else's business in that town, so I said sure I will smoke that with you. And from then on in I tried using pot and other drugs like lsd and mescaline, And we would go out to the Boston harbor islands, and spend all day out there just getting stoned and tripping together, he took photos of the islands and soon started to do more scenic paintings while tripping, and for myself I thought it would help me explore my mind, to get inside and find out why I am me, but I never found any answers and theses drugs out grew their usefulness to me, I am in some of those paintings, there is one of a boy on a ladder in a dirty looking bunker that's me. I must be in over twenty five paintings of his, my sisters are the first real woman he ever painted, and I had become very close friends, he was like the dad I never had, we called him uncle in the family, he got that name just before his alcohol trouble ended, He had gone to the veterans club as he was in the navy, but they told him they didn't want his kind (homosexual) there, get out, And he came to the house in tears, He wanted to commit suicide, no one wanted him he was just a crazy old queer artist, But my mother was there and said Oh no your like family to us we don't care who or what you are, In fact we will call you our "uncle" and he dropped on his knees with clasped hands thanked my mother as he kissed her hand, This was just before I really knew him that well, And was not letting him do portraits of me, that would come soon after this, and his relationship with my entire family and friends soon would completely change his entire life, from being dead from alcohol poisoning soon. To becoming a better and well sought after artist in the latter days of his death, After leaving high school I also spent more time at my grandmother's house in Hingham, in Crow Point my mothers, mother home, my grandfather was there and my mother's brother who also had bought a house across the street and rented it, but stayed at my grandmother's house, he in his time was a scientist for history in the making, he had discovered silicone would store information and that you could retrieve it exactly as you put it in, he discovered what would soon be improved and be called the "microchip", but was only given the patent award from general telephone /Sylvania the company he worked for as a chemical engineer. They took all the credit, as he was working in their lab, he was also involved in Apollo two, the rocket to the moon, it flooded on the launch pad, they called the house to ask my uncle how to remix the gases, which he did and the rocket fired off to the moon, that was so helpful in keeping the momentum going for the race to the moon, Apollo two not getting off the ground would have set us back months, He invented a lens that kept up with the speed of light, so you see what's happening on the moon in real time, But he died young 49, years old of a massive heart attack, and that was going to be a life changing event, to everything the family would end up becoming, and had, he was a collector of fine jewelry, antiques. Artwork sculptures, coins, stamps. And not the lame old cheap stuff it was all the real deal, and he kept it locked in his room and rented sheds, he was a shrewd miser he never gave me a chance, always called me a bad child, He took my sisters everywhere, skiing, camping, boating, I got to go once in a while, but was ignored by him, I never was even given anything to eat or drink while my sisters had the time of their lives, the summers and long weekends off I went over to do the yard work and help my grandparents clean and paint, rake leaves clean house polish furniture, any chore they needed, And became very close to my grandmother again, and there where my father's parents down the road a ¼ mile walk through the woods and behind their home was the highest hill in the area to go up on and get a view of the south shore All you could see where the church steeples rising up out of the tree tops all over the fall time up there was amazing, I would spend many days of my life as a teen, up on that hill, my grandparents lived in Bradley park just off the hill, I loved to visit them and do anything I could to help, the smell of wild flowers where all over daisies and daffodils and tulips, the smell of them always brings me back there as a child looking at all the wild flowers growing in the meadows, and the Honstra farms let their cows wander the hillside, my dad's mom now was just diagnosed with breast cancer, and soon my father's dad would be all alone, it is also where my artist friend came to do many of his paintings. Soon my family left their home in hull just abandoned it! paid what they owed and walked away, breaking even, my mom's mother and her brother where furious, as they had over the years helped them stay in it and would have bought it out right, So we all could have stayed there, or maybe rent it out, but our parents said to keep it quiet, they wanted out of there and quite frankly we all did, though the paranormal activity slowed down a bit, it lingered, in small distractions and in your memories, it was like it took a break but was going to return, and my father's dad was alone and down out right drunk as he could get, a drunk he never would ever recover from and be his demise he was so in love with his wife he cried everyday missing her, And some of it I felt was a lot of guilt, he kept telling her she was not that sick, get up and do your house work your just lazy, I never still to this day would see a man so broken up over a loved one, True love is deeper than we ever can explain and we alone only know it and who it is we feel it for, and if you hurt that one you love and find out you made a big mistake you will grieve heavily more than if you were truly understanding and kind all the way to the end, as this world's spins and twirls and is full of random events and lots of confusion and misunderstandings, if we only just take a minute to stop and take in a nice deep breath, and remember love brought you together in your life, there is always a special person that's keeps you grounded, And focused on who you are and why you need to and want to live, and me where was I ever going to find that,? I need that I want to be in love and be loved back, and that is all I ask, everything else is conditional, and my decision was! To find a girlfriend, A woman and nothing else, that was a goal, and a line I would never cross, and a harder one than I ever imagined, I decided I wanted to live at Crow point with, My mother's mother and the rest of the family moved to Bradley Park, there was not much room in my grandfather's old farm house, and not much either at my mothers, mothers home, So I slept in a room my grandfather built for himself out of a garage, he did all the carvings and wood work by hand, he was an architect and an amazing artist, and carpenter, He was once commissioned by the government to draw important buildings and landmarks all over the world in case they were destroyed in the war and they could be rebuilt. He could run a piece of chalk three feet down a chalkboard and the finest straight rule would not find an error, and take a pencil and a piece of paper and draw a likeness of you, that is shocking to believe someone can do that with such ease, and my grandparents' house was filled with the finest pieces, made by a prominent furniture maker and craftsman my grandfather took special pieces for himself as payment for his help on the books, and drawings he did for the cabinet maker they also along with my uncle went all over the coast of New England in search of antiques, The house was a little museum, everything was dusted and polished, and guess who by, me! I knew every piece of furniture in that house and it was a pleasure to care for such treasures, we were not even allowed shoes on in the house. Because of the oriental rugs that where passed down from her grandparents, But my first two weeks with my grandfather where very frightening. All our lives we were told he was hospitalized for schizophrenia, He had spent twenty five years of his life institutionalized and he did not want me out in his private sanction, the room he built by his own hands, He would get drunk out of his mind with boiler makers for hours, Could he put them down, And he would tell me get out before I kill you, you're not sleeping here, I am coming down with an axe to cut off your head when you sleep, I was so scared I went and told my grandmother, who scolded him right there, he just chuckled, he had no memory of it, she said ignore him, he is harmless, but it continued, and one day his car breaks down an old antique Austin Healy, my grandmother was angry, she said no more tow homes for me that piece of junk is going to the junkyard, and me I had met friends moving to Hingham, Boys originally from Hull, all mechanics and they were teaching me things, I asked my grandmother if I could take a look at the Antique car my grandfather never looked so sad, like his best friend was dead, if he lost that car he would never get over it, she said ok, but if it doesn't run good it's gone, so I look at it, it's never had a wire or spark plug ever replaced not even the points, they were all burnt, and they are telling me it was just tuned up, the distributor must have been original, the mechanic they took it to never bothered to replace any parts, He was just cleaning them putting them back in and making a fortune off my grandparents at 200 dollars, a tune up in 1971, No wonder she wanted to get rid of it, every time they went shopping, they had to get towed home, and where told it's a fussy old antique that requires special attention, and fine tuning constantly, I spent 29 dollars points, plugs wires, cap, and rotor, oil change also, And the car ran till and he drove it until he was so old they had to finally take his license away about 15 years later, never needed a tow again, and we became best of friends, now he had a mechanic, Free, and could keep his car he loved so much, And when they shopped no more tows home, he even let me drive it to high school, I loved it! what a car, I wish I still had it, and my grandfather to this day is my most favorite of people I have ever met, one time I was so scared of him now I miss him so much, His little dog died, it got hit by the milk truck, he grieved for days, and he hand built a beautiful casket, but could not bury the dog, my grandmother came to me and asked I finish, I went out to find him at the grave, he looked at it and said, I keep waiting, hoping he will jump up out of there, I have been waiting for hours, I don't think he is coming back, I took the shovel and I said it's ok, I will help you with this, he stood there watching each scoop of dirt as I placed it on top of the casket, I know he was hoping the sound of the banging of the rocks and dirt would wake up the dog and he would bark so we could rescue him, but it was not to be, he always wanted me to have his car for fixing it for him so he could keep it, but when he died his son said no I can't have it, He never even saw his dad much and had the money to buy ten of them, if he wanted to, and he would not even let me look at it, he towed it quickly away and I never saw it again, Once I asked my Grand Father why he was in a hospital, he said he did not remember even being there, the only memory he had was when they dropped him into a bath tub full of ice and water to shock you back to reality, but once he warmed up he has no recollection of anything else, so he also got lost in that warm blanket of depression only so much further in, than myself, or the treatments now are better, and you may ask why? Why is this person who says he wants to be a girl fix a car? Early in life I was curious how things worked. People seemed sad what they had was broken, and I took everything apart to a point I could put everything back together, and soon I could fix anything after that, I found it made people happy, very happy! They couldn't fix it, but I could, and it was a way of giving a feeling of happiness back. I love fixing things for people, it started with toys, friends toys, I would fix them, I would take them home study them, put them back together and get it to work, How? I don't know, but I would later pass tests in high school as a mechanical genius, and break three records on equivalent tests on the time it took to take them, one I did three times faster than anyone before, and may still hold that record, But high school again,? going back to the ninth grade now, I was two years behind I would not go back, my mother arranged a meeting with a counselor at Hingham high, she said they would have a difficult time bringing me back into school in tenth grade, However We do have a special program called a work study program, and have a lot of kids like yourself who can't keep up, have problems etc., etc., and we would take you in rather than have you not go at all, But you must work and you must show you can come every day, Go to a job you find on your own. And also take tests for up to three hours each day here in class so we can judge you before putting you in your regular classes, So I agreed, my mother wanted me to graduate, why she cared? I don't know! It was more like she just wanted to win; she had brought me to a clinic in Boston two years before to see a group of doctors. They wanted to help my parents find out why I am so depressed and withdrawn in school and failing all my classes, my dad even admits beating me was the only way to get me to understand anything as if I was retarded, He was only there for me as a child for the beatings! If I stepped out of line while he was at work, my mom would say go up and beat your son he needs to be taught a lesson again, I would here his heavy steps come up the stairs real slow and heavy, why he came up so slow I wondered now if he really did not want to come into my room and beat me over a senseless child hood mishap, and that only my mother's word was all that mattered, He never spoke sat and talked about why and maybe next time do this, nothing just the why can't you behave, why did you do that, Then the beating, belts, punches, slaps kicks, I got it all, my sisters could poke me with sticks all day, But if I acted out back I got beating for it, my mother seemed to enjoy the fact she could use those beatings as a way to blackmail me into doing whatever she wanted me to do, And my sisters learned they could push me and bully me also, tease me all day on purpose Even when I asked repeatedly to stop, it would go in one ear and out the next, if they got bored and had me to pick on I had to really be careful or get out of the house, and one of the biggest reasons I did not get a lot of homework done and that got letters sent home which got me more beatings, no one was there, I was all alone, I went more into my own head and locked myself away into my safe little box where I could go away and hide with my little friend and dream away, so they brought me to this clinic I sit with my parents at a big conference table. I am with a group of therapists and doctors and then at the end after they are done talking about me, a doctor says he still needs to see me alone and ask a few more questions, We went to a different office, I was alone with this doctor, who said he had to ask a few more questions and I had no idea it was coming I was kind of surprised, but this was the city, I thought this is what they do in the big hospitals, And it was my first actual "boys" exam, I had never had anyone outside my mother that I know of 'except dad see me, and he asks a few questions about school home, nothing important, then asks that I take my pants down so he can examine me, then just as I am getting ready he asks, do I like being a boy or would you be happier as a girl? And I got suddenly terrified, and so surprised he asked me that, did my parents put him up to this?

Why did he ask me that? I said no! And while I am thinking this he is pulling on my penis lifting my testicles never asked me to cough, that is something I learned later at my next physical exam by a different doctor how different the suburbs are, is all I thought, I felt real strange like electricity shot through me that out of body feeling I used to get at the bus stop, and school hit me, panic attacks, is what they are I would learn more about this condition and need medicine for it when I got older. I was so glad that was over, all the way home my mom said how did you like that doctor she kept saying his name over and over and that he was one of the best there is, but all I could really remember is what he asked me, And that weird physical, and it haunted me daily for the rest of my life. I would never forget that appointment. A doctor asking me out like that made me feel everyone could tell or knew, or was watching me even more, I got so paranoid, and never mind it being my first exam like that ever I was supposed to go back. I think I did a second time and had some more tests, like ink blots and stuff but it was so long ago it all seemed like it all happened in one day, I never went back, a third, I would find out a long time later it was a good thing I did not go back there, The practices done at that hospital where not really medically correct procedures, and the doctor I had do my exam, would later be charged with misconduct, It was too far to travel every day and my parents were not as willing to help as much as they were saying, They put me in a group therapy in Quincy MA, with a bunch of young teenagers with problems but I was too scared! What was I to say?

I felt like I should have been born a woman right there in front of a bunch of other kids, whose worst complaints maybe, they don't get enough television or nights out to party with friends? And mommy and daddy drink too much and fight, they don't get enough love at home, I said nothing and along with my dad not paying the ten dollar co-pay and also if I said anything he picked me up after and would have been the first told, god help me on that ride home, I got kicked out. Some help that was, And it bothered me, there must be help out there, I started to try and find out exactly what it is I need help with, it was by accident at about fourteen I was with my friend Rick, He had just got a pile of old pornographic material from a friend who had to hide it at his house, because his mother found it, I am studying these beautiful woman's bodies I so desire to look like and have and I come upon a little back page story, a story of the first man to be changed into a woman, a transsexual he was called, I read his quick life story up to the decision to change and after the surgery, My god I felt like I was reading about me, There were others, like me, not everything matched perfectly we were from different backgrounds and family, but all the little things that matched, there was a name for this, there are doctor's, it's a medical thing, it is real not made up. But were? I still had my first year in the tenth grade to go through in a whole new school of new faces, All new everything, And what haunted me was that doctor I saw in Boston, He asked me if I wanted to be a girl, He was a doctor did he see something? Did he see through me? Was I feminine in some way that showed? Did my mom know? I was really beginning to think so, and will other people and kids know just by looking?

Again I freeze up more now than ever, if someone even looked at me I couldn't move, I froze like a frightened deer in headlights, it was like I had to force myself to walk while the feeling of electricity shot through my body, just like a mild stun gun the voltage will paralyze you and you can't move, though I never got stunned it has to be similar but less painful. all my horrors of middle school flashed back, I watched how I walked talked, carried my books, dressed, every detail of my own actions I put under a microscope And it was a horrible thing to do, trying to analyze yourself all alone and not knowing what to say and who to say it to. I was so frightened my first year in tenth grade; I don't know how I did it. I should have stayed in ninth in Hingham no one knew me, or not gone back at all. Getting out early for work made it a lot easier, and I made mistakes. I carried my books wrong a lot I held them to my chest, like holding a baby, when I wasn't thinking, boys are supposed to hold them by their side, There where rules, silly little rules,

One morning fooling in a mirror before school I put my hair up in pig tails and put lipstick on, My favorite look! And it was a quick peek I wanted before school that day to help me relax. I remembered to wipe off the lipstick but forgot the pig tails, I went to school with them up, and when I realized what I did, I left them there, I said oh well everyone saw any way why bother, and it looked good on me anyway most of the students did not know who I was, as I walked through the halls, It made that much a difference, Just the classes I went in that knew me, they knew but they just looked no one said anything, a lot of smiles and pointing but that's all, but there where those that looked for that little mistake, that flaw in someone, we know who they are, they are the bullies, I had mine when I was in hull an endless supply of them, all my life, once when I was about ten years old, coming home a block away my house, twenty kids or more stopped me on my way back from Eddie's. A little corner store we all hung out at and played pinball, it was our video game, they were going to beat me, they surrounded me, I ran and got a huge rock and tossed it at them to give me time to escape, they chased me to my house were they told my parents I had thrown a rock at them, and my father grabbed me and beat me in front of all of them, but later realized he made a mistake, He found out I was just defending myself. from a gang of kids ready to beat me, and it was the first time he ever came and said he was sorry, and I was right to defend myself, also a group of guys in hull that followed me into the bathroom almost every morning To kick the crap out of me, it got to a point I never used a bathroom at school anymore, I waited till I got home, and even my toughest of friends were no match for these bullies, they were all way to big and over grown jocks who used their strength to intimidate anyone they wanted, an adult would have had a tough fight with any one of these boys and most were on the football team or hockey some sport and they had political protection to a point, if I had to pee bad enough I walked out of school and found a place to pee on the way home in the woods somewhere, or along the bay, It was good I was on my way out of that town as for a brief moment the town was loaded with guns, they were everywhere kids broke into a collectors house and spread them all over town, soon all the wrong kids on the street had one or more, one even took a shot at a school bus full of kids. The driver thought his bus back fired, he was shooting at someone he thought was a gay kid, it got real crazy, the police where kicking in doors and tearing down walls,

13 kids stood before a judge in front of a complete arsenal of weapons, But by then I was spending more time in Hingham. I was away from hull and its bad way of bringing the worst out of some people. It was so desolate in winter most where summer cottages, seventy five percent of the town emptied on labor day and there was nothing to do, A lot of families on welfare, and large families 10-15 children, and I was not around during that crazy gun spree, I was kind of glad I may have used it on me, if I got my hands on one, but the police found out who had them and got all but a few back, I had found something else I liked, martial arts, I took a course in Shoto Kan watched the new Kung Fu series on television with David Carradine and developed a high interest in that philosophy, and also watched a lot of the Bruce Lee movies and was mostly interested in how he explained what and why he did what he was doing, He was a teacher on film if you really listen, but I soon hated my karate school teacher, he was an arrogant bully. He would never praise me at all, never, he came in and we got beat, the floor was an old bowling ball alley, and nice wood floors. But really waxed and slippery, even when I helped wipe the sweat off the floors with towels, no thank you ever, and if we did not wipe up the sweat we would fall, there where so many in a class you got hit accidently or you hit someone else, and if they told the teacher he wacked you in the stomach, I quit after one year, I told them They give me no incentive to stay, never once did I hear you say you did a little better today keep going, you will improve.

All I got was you are weak and useless why bother coming here, and not just me, he lost a lot of his students, But! The philosophy and the whole idea of a chi, a Ying and a yang, sounded real to me I understood the feel of it, and the technique behind the punch to make it more powerful, it really worked, it was a method of physics, using circles and leverage for strength, there had to be a real good school somewhere and someday I would learn more about it, I did many years later. a normal person hits with the weight of their arm, this teaches you how to get all your weight of your body into the area the shape of your hand and release into the body where it has to go and disrupt everything inside even damaging internal organs, but I still had to get through high school I thought it would be easy just pop in a couple hours then out to a job but the new faces everywhere. They all felt like they were all staring at me, I pushed through what seemed to me a sea of blank faces with big eyes every morning like those kissing fish, in fish tanks with the big eyes that just stare at you, and went into a class full of kids who were half retarded, Or they were there because they never cared or neither did their parents, This meant absolutely no life in school, I could not socialize with anyone in the normal classes especially in Hingham, it just meant I had to be even more reclusive and alone, I smoked pot every morning before school, and kept a happy little buzz on while I was there, or I never could have made it, Marijuana gave me a very nice feeling, I felt peace and happiness, I wondered how close it was to femininity! and really believed I used it to induce the feelings of feeling feminine, or just feeling good, I had no other real feelings any more, just depression, happiness was as brief as the smile of the moment.

My high became my female emotion inside. and not as a personality but as a feeling, I had only experienced a lot of sadness, disappointment, anger, frustration, fear, doubt, not a lot of happiness and I always thought of femininity as happiness, Pot gave me a feeling I could not bring to the surface myself, finally I get a job, working for the for administration building working for the office of teaching services, My boss was a straight out guy follow the rules, My name always starts with mister, do what I say and we will get along, He was tough, he wanted a lot of work done. No breaks! work every minute you are there, and I challenged him a lot to find me work, I always knew he meant well and only was there to help troubled kids like myself make it, I took all his criticism and worked with the department till I graduated, we actually became good friends at work and well trusted each other, He later hired my sister, he asked when he saw the last name on her application if we were related she said yes, and he said that's enough for me, you are hired, Everyone in the Hingham school department administration building, from the school superintendent to the maintenance man where the greatest people I would ever get to work with, and to this day I hold the fondest memories of my life from there in that time, I go to the fourth of July parade every year, And I sit near the building I worked at One of my favorite memories is leaving work to come home to my grandmothers at school vacation week, it was the Christmas weekend holiday. and opening the big old 150 year old double doors that night to go home to my grandmothers, And seeing the biggest snowflakes, I ever to this day have ever seen so slowly floating down onto the old Hingham Square,

It took me back hundreds of years in that moment, the town looked like it has for the last two hundred years or more. It is all historical land marks, Lincolns grandfather log cabin was walking distance near were a statue of Lincoln himself is immortalizes, and beside me the first church to be built from the 1600's, The large snowflakes where so big and heavy as they gently drifted down looking like little angels floating down from heaven, as hard as my own struggle was, I was ok there in that moment And moments I had like that to put away in my memory and treasure always breathe life into me when I need it, It made me feel I could do this and feel hope of a future, as I go along through this pain and life I have become so confused in, I have hope that a wonderful moment awaits around the corner, and myself for now, I could tell no one, but I felt so good that day watching the snow fall. If I could ever travel back in time, for just a few moments that's one place where I would go, the strong feelings of suicide as a teen where my worst, every day I woke up with the very first vision in my mind of hanging myself by the neck, I still would have to go into that school and see all those kids. And the girls, the ones who try and get your attention, they know your name, but you don't know there's! so you know they are interested in you, some are so beautiful when I look at them I freeze, and it's not that silly boy shyness that we watch on television shows, like American pie, or animal house, it's absolute fear, real fear of rejection, but not the rejection most boys would face, mine is different, it's real! It is going to happen 99.9999 percent of the time I would try. and be devastating emotionally, even life changing, to a point of committing suicide telling the wrong girl, who would take it wrong and tell everyone I know, I always wanted to be honest and up front fast, I knew any girl I would go out with, it would only be a matter of time before I would tell her how I really felt, And just not to break up but I was so eager to find out if anyone wanted someone like me. Every day when I walked home from work, I walked right buy a dress shop in the middle of town, Cante's Dress Shop. They displayed all there real best beautiful dresses in the windows. I usually glanced and kept walking, if I felt safe stopped and dared look at only few seconds, And every girl in school who said hello or showed an interest in me or I was interested in and I wanted so bad to talk to, I would see myself in one of those dresses with her, Still! just like I was doing as a young child, it had not changed it was still the same, only more romantic, as I would imagine myself with her on a bench or a nice soft green lawn in a park, somewhere explaining myself waiting for the rejection or hoping I would get a big hug. and be told everything will be ok, but I never did, I never had the courage, I only knew what crying was like and this was my year to cry, when I lived with my grandmother in Hingham I had three pillows, on a good night I soaked through one and a half but usually and most nights I went through all three. Till I got to the very last pillows last dry side and hoped it would stay dry enough to get me through the night, if not I would need a towel which meant no sleep that night, And not many of them I would sleep at all but maybe an hour, I would lay there and just cry all night long, soaking my pillows right through, once those pillows where a suicide device, I put one over my face and clasped my hands behind my head real tight to suffocate myself until I saw a bright blue spark and then it just went dark, when I became aware again there was a lot of fear to open my eyes to see where I was, I was so scared, heaven or Hell it could be either one or that I was still at home, The only other time, I would try would be about a month later, I took powerful horse tranquilizers and ground them up, and snorted them up into my nose, I could not move, I was completely paralyzed, only my eyes could move, my grandmother had just gone out, when I started and in what seemed like ten minutes she was back, I could hear the banging of pots and pans as she prepared dinner, five hours had just gone by in what seemed like only minutes, I started to be able to move a finger and soon was able to get up and recover real slowly, If my grandmother had come out and seen me she would have called an ambulance, I would have frightened that poor woman, I was so glad she never came out to see me, I have never made another attempt since, it is a very scary experience to "fail" at. and I did not really want to hurt the inside part of myself it was the outside I did not like, but I would hurt the inside part of myself hurting the outside, It helped me to think like that now, I have decided to seek more help in prayer, and help from god, my grandmother is very religious and catholic, and is a very strong influence in my religious beliefs, she has priests visit often at the house for tea, and not so much that I want to follow a type of religion but she is a woman. I have come to trust and admire so much, But I feel if I was born correct, I may have been a nun, and I know my grandmother would have put me right into school for it, if I asked her, And what I have already seen in my own life I know we go someplace when we die, But I was very depressed and was planning a third attempt, which I could not help doing, as much as I want to live and make it and be here for gods purpose I feel I just don't belong here, and I am not wanted, by anyone and some of my prayers are god will take me in my sleep away from here and I won't wake up too this anymore.

And I still do, I still have those days so bad I cry myself to sleep and pray I will be taken that night, I had to be patient and keep trying, But I also wanted to die, In eleventh grade they put me in regular classes, I sat next to this real pretty blonde girl named Linda, we became friends at school, And I tried to build a relationship with her outside of school, But I was so damn scared of the rejection and the horrible consequences that may follow, if I told her how I really felt, not just hurting myself but her also, I could not get passed her innocent smile, and eventually I gave up, I did have dinner with her family once and we went out a couple times but I knew just by becoming too close to anyone, that I was going to tell them, I did not want to keep this hidden I want it right out fast, if I am to get dumped do it and get it over with, finding that strength is very hard, And not only getting dumped but everyone they will tell why they dumped me, and it's my own conscious that bothers me so, I feel the pain of hurting others more than myself, it is my weakest point of my personality, but I cannot find the strength to be hard, and if I hurt a person inside I feel it back so much harder and it will haunt me forever, one day it will come, thanked me for telling them, I did not know how to get any relationship even started without hurting someone, I just stopped seeing her, vanished from her life, When I was fifty years old I sent her a letter and apologized for disappearing like I did, and explained why I did to her and a few others I did the same, I just vanished from their lives with no explanation, They all understood and wrote back and where happy for still remembering them, and I was so happy they remembered me, I took a chance they even would, and still being concerned about what I had done to them and need not apologize, they asked I Just be brave and they wished me luck, I had just moved back with my parents and was back and forth a while, I had been asked to come back, by my mother, I don't know why! My younger brother moved into my room at my grandmother's house and, I went over to Bradley Park. I mostly kept to myself, I tried to date a couple more times but they were all disasters one after the other, I could not get my male role model right, whatever it was I was supposed to do and how I was supposed to act, I got it wrong, always, one of my biggest mistakes always was waiting too long to kiss, or put my arm around her, I always was afraid and I know she may have felt I did not like her, but I did, any one woman I approached I wanted to honestly love, not just use, and all I ever felt was I was hurting others along with myself, I cannot bare hurting anyone and making them feel pain I really began to feel this is it, I am going to be alone for the rest of my life, and looked at a tree at the top of bakers hill to put a rope on to hang myself, I wanted a nice last view, it had to be just the right spot. And so someone could find me and not let wild dogs eat me, And it's true to this day, I walk this alone, find many, many loved ones, but, you yourself may face many times in your life you are the only one in your life that's going to reach in and pull you back up, others are all around to help but this is so hard they don't have any idea what you are going through. unless they are just like you, and you cannot explain your pain 100 percent, It's just you against the world, and you will win if you don't let those who don't want you to win get to you, and there are a lot of them, and those that love you are frightened by the outside forces that hate you, and some are to be afraid to stand out and say no, I love this person, I found a mental health clinic to go to in Quincy Ma, I was given the head doctor, after I told the receptionist why I wanted help, that poor old woman never looked so surprised, I told him how I felt right away, He had never even heard of this it seemed, A man in a woman's body? He asked that's how you really feel? And asked questions for several sessions about three and at the end threw his hands up and sorry I cannot help you I think what's really wrong with you, is that you are just gay, a homosexual, and afraid to admit it, go find a boyfriend or try to find your own kind out there, whatever that may be, just don't come back here, I was totally shocked, I wanted to go home and hang myself right away, the bus ride home was planning and preparing my last details, But all I could see was his foolish grin when he threw me out, I would not give him that satisfaction, that day, Then A day in the school lunch room cafeteria that's a revelation and such a surprise to me. As I am sitting at my table a kid sits beside me, He is so familiar, I know this kid, I have seen him hundreds of times, he lived in the old neighborhood I grew up in when I was five years old and under, in Worlds End Hingham Ma, My mother would come back to the old neighborhood to visit the friends she made. We would come back and hang around and play in the old places we used to, He was my mother's friends neighbors kid, I said are you so and so from worlds end and he said yes and I know who you are too, you're the boy who wanted to be a girl, we all came down to your yard when we were kids to beat the shit out of you, you must have been like 2-4 years old then, and he just said nothing after that, he went back to eating his lunch like nothing happened, I didn't say anything either, I was in shock hearing that! and right in front of about ten other kids, who all just stared at me, I swear I nearly slid right off my seat, was I embarrassed, and not only that! It hit me how far back all this went, I didn't even remember that, I was too young, but 5 and 7 year old kids did, and that meant my parents also knew something too. A lot of people did! I must have been punished very early in life to never be like or act out like a girl. Or I would be beating or punished, there was always such an element of fear and that I was doing something wrong when I cross dressed before anyone ever told me it was, when I was a young child, It felt wrong like I was stealing, but when I stood there and looked at myself I felt right, it is so confusing and it has been this way for ever. But now I was beginning to understand, A little more anyway, why the guilt and also why it's there still. And how far back this battle has gone on, and what may have happened to those nice toys I had and who really smashed them up, It may not have been me, but those boys who came to beat on me that broke all my toys, so much flooded my brain the day he sat and told me that, My mother was in a constant struggle with my boyhood, or manhood. She praised me as her son, she told me the world was mine as a man I was told if anything happened to my father she would need me the most, I would be the one who takes over, she put me on a tall pedestal of gold, any time I looked sad or depressed I was told I could tell her anything, I was the son she always wanted, she always put that in, I could never tell her I felt like I wanted to be her daughter, it was unfair she said that every time, It stopped me from telling her, what I really needed to tell her, and I think it was on purpose and she always made sure my hair was cut, Soon as it hit my ear it was time to cut it, and I hated it, I did not want my hair cut, I admit, I got conned, Father and son dress alike day, go off to the barber shop, learn to be a little man stuff, there was an element of fun to it, I got to hang out with dad, just us two. Being with dad I always felt proud and invincible But there were not many of those days, He worked a lot and soon retired to watching sports and drinking liquor at night and we lost touch, and my mother, she wants that haircut, buy 14 years of age, it has become unbearable to cut it anymore, every time I had to sit in that chair A little voice inside was crying for help, I am a girl, I want my hair long!!! but those words could not ever come out, they froze on the edge of my lips, It was my little friend in her box yelling out, but could not be heard, as I felt my mom's satisfaction of pushing that clipper through my head, and always saying good! you won't look like a little girl now, my dad he stood there and made sure I did not move a muscle or he would slap me right back in that chair, and one day it just happened it got too long, The Beatles arrived I had an excuse, everyone else is, my parents refused, it was get in that chair, and the beating to make me started, my mother promises she will just take off a little. She says she knows how the kids now are growing it longer and understands, and she will just take a little bit off, and starts out ok, taking little snips, but then I feel that clipper get jammed into my head and I just snapped, I pushed her away and ran upstairs. looked at myself all hacked up in the mirror, "my mother was no barber", and I heard my dad coming up to give me a beating, I tore the mirror off the wall ran to the top of the stairs and as hard as I could, I threw the whole medicine cabinet down at my dad just missing him, he ducked, the force of the cabinet was so hard it scared him, He said you could have killed me, he said you know what? If you want your damn hair! keep it, I am done fighting over this, and he left me alone, I was surprised, we became better friends again, there was such a long period of silence between us, I could count on one hand how many times we did something together. I hoped for better, but he was a prejudice man, on his way to work and home he would be harassed by blacks even getting full beer bottles thrown at him. while he tried to go into work every day to provide for his family, He used to get off at the train station and walk about a quarter mile to work, I went with him a few times to work on a Saturday, there were signs that said no spitting, he said those are only meant for the blacks they are the only ones who come in and spit, they are dirty and we will get germs from them, and bums sleeping under cardboard boxes, begging for change for their liquor. While he worked for his, My second oldest sister married a black guy, We never told him, we told him he was French, He fooled him because his mother was white so it worked, but he had to wear a baseball cap when he came to the house, he had the natural African American hair, But the way he was never reflected on me I was never prejudice, how could I be, here I am one of the most hated kind on the planet, Everyone hates me even gay people don't understand or accept me to well, they to, like that doctor I saw think I am one of them in denial, in third grade the first black family moved to town and I was one if his first friends, He used to come to play at my home, and I used to go to his house to visit, but he got pneumonia and died He played outside one day to long, He had never seen snow before like we had and could not bring himself inside to warm up, He was just having too much fun, but I know what people say about someone like me, I have learned all the slang, all the hate words, all the feelings of hate and that killing someone like me would do the world a favor, and it's hard, you have days you are so depressed. You start to feel these people are right, you don't have a right to exist, you should just die, or be killed, what are you anyway, I have trouble eating I feel I don't deserve it, I want to push it away and it won't go down, I fill up quick, you're not really a man, you're not really a woman, you're in between a kind of what you have to call an "IT" because you will neither be one or the other to them, you will always just be in between, an "IT" Never ever getting to ever be completely just one, to them they will always say, what is "IT"? And to me that word is the same as being called the "N" word. A word we no longer use any more, because as a people we have grown and have learned what a hurtful word it is, and there are other words we are no longer using when we refer to a group of people or any individual different from the rest of us, that hurts so deep inside, and for people like myself the word IT is very painful, A cause of feelings of depression and loneliness in anyone who goes into this transition, or have a feel of knowing you don't belong, and they never go away, to become the woman you know you are, then you will do it, Even in the face of the entire worlds rejection, If you could just have your one day of your life as who you really are before you die, you're going to know it was all worth it. But the time you spend becoming who you are and the pressure from those around you to stop you, are very tiring and very overwhelming and they will remain with you forever. Like hounds on your trail, they will never leave you alone, you have to remove yourself from them, They will always want you to stop and go back, Even your own doubts that you will have from time to time, as you age, but it all comes back to who you are, and your real identity, and no matter how you dress it, turn it, grow hair on it, express it, your body is just the outside part everyone sees, they don't see inside, your soul, especially when it's so hidden, and afraid, and you are so afraid to be who you are and you know you could be killed for it. And to show what is hidden inside, you have to dress your outside self in the gender that you are, so if they know who you were before, once you do, and they know. They won't forget, Eleventh grade comes and soon I would meet my first love and I mean it "that one", the one you never forget or get over, ever! I was about to have the two most happiest years of my life and have someone I would know as a close intimate friend to this very day still, I would meet her with my old hull neighborhood close friends, we had drove to hull for old times, I was glad to get out and was recovering from the suicides I just tried and was planning another, Three girls we all knew and soon met up with and got together with in the car sat and talked, Soon we had an arm around each girl, it was quick, I was scared as hell but I didn't want to be the one who didn't! I was shocked that she snuggled up to me, I never in my life thought a girl as beautiful as this would ever come near me, I knew her from school, I had remembered her from my first year of the fourth grade just before they took me out for that ear surgery, I was in line between classes my friend Rick yells over, hey look, that's my cousin, they just moved to hull, I look up and there is this beautiful little girl, In a plaid jumper, white blouse, long dark curly hair and round large brown eyes waving and smiling at "me"! I couldn't take my eyes off her, She just took the whole hall way up, I just stood there and watched in awe as she walked by with the rest of her classmates, I just crushed completely out, I stopped breathing for a minute or two, I have to say one thing is that I always had healthy crushes, I loved girls, I even had a crush on Wendy the witch. The comic book character, but it was also that I wanted to be like her do the nice little magic tricks to help people like she did, But I would not see this girl again except occasionally, I would see her playing with the neighborhood kids and sometimes playing with her cousins and my sisters; When they came to visit, But right now here she was again sitting beside me and my arms around her and a feeling of everything I was feeling about my gender drift away, it wasn't on me as heavy, I was relaxed more than I thought, It was as if this is what I needed all this time, I only hoped at that moment I would see her again and I did, we dated a couple weeks it was wonderful and she is so beautiful, But my gender inside is always reminding me who I am, and my own promises to myself to always tell the truth, have caught up with me, we were together on a couch hugging, she said she was unhappy at home at the time, and was having some troubles there, kids things, but at the time when we are young they seem like monsters to us, I said it's ok nothing you are going through are as bad as any of my troubles, and she said, what? I said, I can't say, at the moment, it's very bad anyway, and I am afraid you won't like it or me anymore if I tell you what is really bothering me, she says, you can tell me anything, anything at all, it's ok, don't worry, I promise if you do, it will just be between you and me, and will always be like this, Anything we say is between us always, (a promise she has kept), so I look quickly into her impatient eyes all sparkling and full of life, and I feel safe, I say all my life, I felt like I should have been born a girl, and she froze, she did not move a muscle I just felt her grip me tight. She did not take one breath, I was so scared, God what have I just done? she is about to get up, run for her life and tell my two closet friends who are right there at the home, I grew up with, I was a freak, but, then she just relaxed, didn't say anything, we were both quiet, she looked at me and smiled, that was good, When we said goodnight I got a real nice soft wonderful kiss, but was sure it would be the last, and it wasn't, we went back out again, I never brought it up again to her I just enjoyed every minute with her I had, I never thought of anything else, within weeks I fell totally in love and being anyone or any particular sex at the time meant nothing as long as I was with this woman I was with, She was a gem!! her eyes had a wonderful sparkle to them and a smile that drew you in close, my soul just melted into hers when we held hands, I loved holding her hands so much, I felt as if, I had become a complete person for the first time ever in my life, I was completely in love and a love I would never get over! ever, The only important thing to me was to do everything I could to make sure I always saw that wonderful smile and that sparkle in her eyes when she came to greet me, sadly though we parted ways after a couple years only we never said goodbye, she said I never want to say that, and I did not either, we said, see you later, when I knew I would not be with her any more my soul felt like it just pulled back inside of itself and became cold, there was a chill to it, it would never again reach out to anyone else again, although It tried, I never ever felt I had a soul mate again, Or I was just too afraid to let myself have one, losing one hurts to much, a year into our relationship I did something awful I would regret for ever, I betrayed myself and this woman I loved so much. what seemed like a simple act was not, It was a moment of doubt, and stupidity, I had beautiful long blond hair, it took years to grow it, it was waist long, I was very proud of it, it was my female side, and it was my own secret, But it had started coming out of style, I was getting called a freak daily, people in cars stopped and stared, yelling hey you a boy or a girl constantly, I felt paranoid everywhere I went, Hingham was a town of rednecks, and one day I let it all get to me, seemed that day like everywhere I went I got harassed, stared at, Old ladies clutched their pocket books and scurried along, I went into a barber shop and said give me the regular, and off it came, all of a sudden I felt naked, I looked at myself and was shocked I was no longer myself, I had just become what everyone else wanted me to be, and the worse was to come when I go and see the closest one to my heart, she is shocked and mad, and angry, that I would do that without telling her, and she was so right, to be so mad. Here was my other half, my soul mate, the only woman on the planet I felt I was one with, complete with, when we held hands I felt my soul just flow into hers and become warm, just as if I was a piece cut out of a puzzle and found my matching part, If anyone was to change anything on my body it should only have been her, how wrong I was to betray my soul and hers, as it was attached to me, and her also, I had just hurt the person I loved more than anyone else in my entire life, With a foolish act, at a weak moment, I should have called her, I had no idea how to amend such a horrible mistake, and with all things a pair of scissors and clippers, just like when my own mother ripped my soul to pieces as a child, I had just done it to myself, And I felt homely and could not even look at myself at all, how could she now, I was that monster in the mirror people will say I am going to turn into, every time I looked at myself, I cannot look in mirrors even today, being thought of as a monster all your life affects you, And sometimes looking into a mirror I see that monster everyone else sees, A lot of times today my wife says what! Are you conceited! Always looking at yourself like that! When I put my makeup on and do my grooming, and check myself before I go out, and she is so wrong, I am so scared when I look at myself, most of the time I see the scary monster everyone else sees, and I just hope I make it through the day, Soon she came to me one day and said she thought we should both see other people and not stay as a couple at this time, I felt it was coming but to hear it was a reality more than I could have ever been prepared for, like a death, I cried so hard I could not let her go, but I did, and cried for days and as I was alone. And again in touch with my feelings all to myself, That's when I realized I would never be the same again, I searched through my heart and mind all through my emotions and pain, all my mistakes, what I could have done to lose this wonderful woman and this beautiful moment I just had, So if I ever fell in love like that again I would be more careful and never make any mistakes, and never hurt someone who loves me, Or anything that would cause me to have lost this wonderful moment and woman I had in my life, All my happiness shattered like glass on a coldest of winters day, my emotions as fragile as a dry leaf you can crumble easily in your hands, and just blow away, I learned that when you love some like that you never leave them out in even the minor of decisions you will make in your life, or you are not one, you are by yourself incomplete, half a person, and my life had a purpose to make myself complete, also I did not become angry or look for a way to hurt with force, or make threats of violence if she dare seek anyone else, I only wanted her to be happy more than myself, I turned inwards more it's not like saying she just came out of me, it was me going in, and I had learned and had just experienced feelings I never in my life had dealt with before, very emotional ones, and each one I pulled off and studied like the petals of a flower to be explored after it is taken from its branch, when I realized I was not handling this situation like a man but I was handling it like a woman. And wanting to grow from what I have just experienced, not to run out to bars and grab another woman to forget the pain I was in, as many of my peers did and do and said I myself should. I had a girl I worked with that flirted with me all the time and the drinking laws where eighteen not twenty one and still had the phone number of the nice blonde girl Linda in Hingham that wanted to see me still, And more than all of them I remembered my little friend I had in my little safe box I had pushed away and forgotten she was still there, patiently waiting, as if expecting me to return, and I went to her again she brought me to places in my mind that comforted me at a time I was so lost and she helped me heal, And from here, to looking finding a place for myself somewhere, she was hope, she made no promises but she gave me that little bit of hope where at this moment now I had none at all, The one love I just had and lost, was to be forever in my heart, to be cherished, and not to ever be embraced and held again warmly in my arms I would not feel it's warmth again but only the memory of that moment when I remembered her, though not as good, at least what I held once so close to me I would cherish forever, I would light a little candle in my heart to keep me warm and to remember her always and what love felt like so I would know if I had found it again, if I ever could, and I would make sure I would do anything I had to, to never lose it again. or never hurt it or scare it again and make it want to leave me, I don't believe that to many men would go into their own hearts this way as I do, it was a rebirth of myself, that she was here to stay. And that the part of me that was alive was just beginning to grow, I had realized at that moment I was truly a woman, it took an extreme emotional change to bring out that feeling that I would have forever, and I promised myself I would never push her away and keep her hidden from myself again, And if she had been with me I may not have made the mistakes I made that destroyed this wonderful moment that I may never have again, I did not think I would ever see her again, I just lost her forever, she was away about 3-4 months and she called and wanted to see me again, and we went back out, I felt so happy and was still so in love, I enjoyed every minute of our last months we would have, But it had a feeling of not being as it was I could not get this feeling I had like before, I had changed, I loved her as much as ever before and never wanted it to end, but there was a sadness to myself only I could feel, every time I looked at her a voice inside me said "tell her", "tell her," It haunted me daily, I wanted so bad to tell her, all about my feelings and I wanted her to see me dressed as a woman, I wanted also to let her see this soul inside I hid, it had been years since I had myself, it would have been so exciting to me if I allowed myself to let her see this nice kind friendly person I was hiding all alone inside, but I was leaving soon and did not want to scare her away, I wanted to spend every last precious minute I had with her and not lose one second of any of them. My soul felt like sand in an hour glass falling through its hole waiting for the end to come, which I knew was going to arrive when a plane ticket with air force on it said time to go, I had changed in those moments and I wanted to tell her more now than ever, it hung on the end of my lips every time we saw each other, I hoped that she too might share that side of me, though not so much as to come along physically as much as to come along emotionally to give me strength, but I could not, I wanted not to harm her or take a chance at this moment and risk never to see her again, when I knew soon we would part. and I know that what I had said about my gender had to be in the back of her mind somewhere, The thought of ever hurting or bringing any hurt to her again would only come back at me even more, I had to go on a journey all alone, No matter how many people I would meet or touch in my life time no one would ever fill that empty place in my soul, and my heart that was full of her love, she was in there forever I kept her and all her memories like anyone else who has that first and only love does, Locked it up to embrace till the end of time, that we may someday see each other again, and if I have become a woman I am hoping that she remembers me well and can still tell her I love her still just as much now as I did then and I will never stop, and always the hope of me ever once again in my life just to say hello again, it's me, can we talk,? The year following year was my lost year, I gained nothing, and lost everything I had, along with my soul, the recruiter was all over me calling me constantly, He told me I joined and signed my life to the government and had to go, but all that I would find out what a lie that it all was, But I really wanted and needed to do was to heal a knee injury and I needed surgery I tore the one of the two ligaments that hold your knee in place they look like an X the anterior ligaments My parents had no health insurance for me I was eighteen, I wanted to be a police officer and get my training in the air force, and I went in and did the worst of it. and was doing good I had about 9 days left, the worst was over but suddenly my knee gave out every time I stepped off a sidewalk I fell, and found out that my recruiter sent me in at the wrong time, there was no police training school for another 18 months He lied, he made fifty bucks for everyone he sent in, He made no contract with me at all, He just said he did, and when he said I had to hurry and get on the plane for my school, there was no school to go to, it was all being done at Texas, all the contracts and agreements where being done as I sat in an office when they found out I had not picked any career.

And all they gave me where jobs like picking up trash, cooking, kitchen help, all meaningless jobs, I was disappointed all that work for nothing, and that the schools where for new recruits as an enlistment incentive, I hope they all were better at reading the recruiter than I was, and the eighteen month wait was no guarantee there would be a training spot open for me and I would most likely have to reenlist, to get one,

I was so lied to by my recruiter I was allowed to break my contract, which I did, I actually never really had one, it was a mess down there, my T. I. Said go back to Boston and slap him for us, I would have stayed if they sewed up my knee and let me heal but they said no! it's an injury you did before you joined, And my parents just said I was a failure and just a dropout, don't come back here, we don't want you, What a lonely feeling homelessness is when it is so suddenly dumped in your lap, and you find your family rejects you before you even tell them you're looking for help for this type of problem. And after that, I went to California with the money I had for what I had already earned and just changed my ticket. and lived on and off with my two older sisters for about a year but I never felt that welcome buy their husbands even though I paid rent, I felt like I was intruding, And I never slept well I had the same dreams every night over and over, And I dreamt them every night for over ten years, That I was walking through deserts, looking at tumble weeds blowing around, And knocking on doors asking for her, and no replies just looking out at the empty deserts again those old houses in old western ghost towns, I would see their hands, bodies, and heads even their hair, but never their faces as they pointed outwards and when I turned back to look and say where? I don't see anyone! they were gone, the people and old houses would disappear, and fade into the wind and sand blowing through the empty hills, I cried myself to sleep every night, I just turned over on my side and wept so my wife would not see me, I felt cut in half. I knew I was going to feel alone for the rest of my life and, In my life at that moment I believed it was just her I looked for but also later I realized her presence and her appearance was burned in my memory forever and she represented love to me, and the only I ever had, and I lost it, and I had so foolishly let it fall from my hands Like all that desert sand blowing through the hills of those empty deserts. I was walking through, and that's what those dreams meant, they are my search for love, being so alone and no one to be in love with, no one to tell them I love you and really feel it, I need that, I live for the feeling that I need to love someone so much and make them so happy they want to love me back, I always feel I scare everyone away, I did not have much money out there jobs where hard to keep, lots of layoffs, I worked as a tool and die maker apprentice on and off but U.S steel eventually went on a big strike there was nothing for work, Ronald Regan was the Governor, and if you weren't born in California, or Mexican, they treated you like you came from another country, you were picked last for jobs, girls out there, I tried to go out with backed away, some giggled and laughed.

They said they felt I was to gentle, they felt like they were in bed with another woman, that surprised me, that rejection hurt more than any I ever had and was embarrassed by it, Or they were shallow and fast and rude not what I was use to back home, If you didn't have a way to take care of them and spend a lot of money on them they would not even talk to you, I didn't know what to think about that, I didn't get or want many returns, Especially the surprise of being to gentle. that was always a hurtful surprise it has made me very afraid to approach woman, It will be something in my future that I will have the hardest time overcoming, When I get the most important part of my soul hurt I will pull myself away for a very long time until the fear of contact again frightens me, I sought help out in San Francisco, thinking the gay community hotlines would know something, and find me a place to get the help I needed, I went in on a train one day, a woman was on the train on the aisle beside me, she was very beautiful, she reminded me a lot of someone I had just left behind, a group of men became loud and started talking about their sexual encounters the night before, but not with woman, they talked about being with other men, It was foul and disgusting to hear talk like that so open on a public train, A lipstick rolls down the aisle and a guy runs down to pick it up, it was a gimmick to get a peek! At me! I got sick at that point, and at the next stop I got off, so did the woman, I waited for the next train and watched down the track, I pay no attention to what was going on around me, a train came and the door opened, I look! the woman who had gotten off was now getting back on, she had gotten off the train for the same reason as me, To escape those gay men and their horrible talk of their activities, She looked at me and smiled, she knew I must be straight and preferred woman and that part she was so right, and I was so tempted at that moment to approach her or at least talk, But I could not bring myself to it, I felt that I would only come to the same ending I had just come from before and lose another loved one, I heard also if you are a straight guy in Frisco a woman will support you because it has become so hard to find a straight guy, but I would never do that and it would have been a lie, as much as she would have been my only partner, I dare not ever say what I really felt like, the incident with the gay men actually made a impasse' between any relationship with her, it ruined it, she would only assume the worst to come. and I was just some gay guy using her, what a mess, she looked too nice to hurt, any woman is too nice to hurt, and I don't want to bring any hurt into anyone else's world. now but my own, A need to search for who I am now was important and I had nothing to offer, If I had a way to support myself at that moment I would have tried, and I if I did and had to tell her I do not think that she would ever understand and how could she, I myself don't, All this was so hard, and all this went through my mind in between just a few stations, as the train moved towards the city of San Francisco, I wanted an end to all this, why did I feel like two people where part of me fighting for control, and only one can win. Who helps you? How do I make myself feel like a complete person and without another person with me, like a soul mate, I don't want to be alone! It was even harder than I thought it would be, no matter how brave I told myself I had to be, it was harder than I even imagined, I wanted to be in love again with someone, But there was no one for me, who would want me? I was so lucky once in my life to have had someone I loved so much. And I knew I may never again, I had to do this alone, I had to become a complete person on my own, and the struggle was just beginning, At the age of 20 thinking back you would think the worst of it was getting behind you, the horrible teen years, But in no way was it, it was just beginning, I got in touch with a hotline and was told to meet with a person named Jack, I got his number and arranged an early evening appointment, we were to meet at a restaurant near a rail station, I am early I was told where to sit and I told jack what color jacket I would wear so he knew it was me, In walks this older man in coveralls, looked like he just got off the night shift as a janitor or machine shop tech, we introduced each other and as the waiter filled our glasses with water he loudly asks, so how long have you been cross dressing? That just completely surprised and embarrassed me, I had no idea he would say that so openly and that loud and in front of so many people, But hung I in there I thought it must be a safe place he knows of, or he would not have asked like that, we talked briefly and he said well now I am going to show you the world you so eager seek, are you ready? I said ok, And we stopped at a home, A couple lived there a man and his wife, we spoke briefly, they called jack Nancy, I was directed into a room and shown some art work for about ten minutes and then asked to return to the table, and there was a woman sitting there, It was jack, She had changed clothes makeup wig everything, in minutes, a completely different look, I was amazed I never saw anything like that ever, a feeling of not being so alone came over me, I was with someone going through the same thing I was going through, it was amazing. She took me around to all the clubs in town that others like us went to, it opened a world to me I never knew about, they were beautiful, many of them, and somewhere not so, you could tell right away they were men, but they had a lot of heart, they gave it their all to be the lady they so wanted to be, I had several meetings with Nancy but they became fruitless she insisted that if I was to go on a hormone program and meet the doctors that provide them\I would have to get by her first, what did she mean,? She was no doctor, or therapist, she is just another transsexual in transition no real credentials, just a lot of friends out there, And I begin to realize that she is expecting sexual favors from me, to prove I can handle being a woman before she will introduce me to her doctors. I was hurt, I came for help, I came to find doctors, I did not think someone going through what I was, would put up such a wall for me to climb if I wanted help, I stopped seeing her and again felt alone and scared, And the first thought to myself was, this must be what that first doctor in Quincy Ma. Thought would be a good idea, well I guess not, I hope he reads my book, I can't remember his name just that it had a lot of x, y and Z's in it, I hope you read this and see how long I have struggled and how closed a mind you have, and that I hope that you're not still telling patients you don't know what to do with, to go find their own kind, it's not good therapy. And I also said to myself this so called Nancy she is not like me at all! She is not half the woman I am, she did not pass "my" test. She turned on her own, hoping only for her own gain, and maybe some sexual adventures from a scared lonely person to take advantage of, and left someone frightened and alone out in the cold instead of saying yes! I will help you! I know a therapist that will get you started, then she calls my home where I rent a room in a private home in San Leandro and in a deep male voice told them it was Nancy, they all looked at me real weird when I got off the phone. They said some guy calling himself Nancy is on the phone, And then I heard them saying things about me like oh my god he is gay, I was horrified. I called him back and said thanks I have to move right out, I just lost my home, these people are old and don't understand, and by now all my unemployment was just about gone. I was homeless I had slept in a shelter a few times, once off the street in the woods, a friend let me have a room in his house for a few months, This time I called my grandmother for help and this time, I could come home, my dad was very sick, He was dying from alcohol poisoning, greyhound had a special, Travel anywhere in the country for 76 dollars for the bicentennial year 1976, I got a ticket and headed home on a 56 hour nonstop ride on a bus, when I got to Boston there was snow everywhere, I had forgotten how to walk on it, and I must have fallen twenty times before I got from the bus stop to home, and that hurts, I was welcomed in, everyone was happy to see me, I took one look at my dad and was horrified, he was all yellow, all over, The whites of his eyes, skin, all yellow! it was January, he would die the following year in February, 77, I got up every morning lit the fire in the fire place cooked everyone there breakfast, made sure there was more firewood, It was the only heat the house had, and I had to go out into the woods and cut my own, but it was nice wood, cedar trees fell all over the ground. the other trees out grew them and wiped most of them out, all I had to do was drag them home And they cut like butter and smelled so good, and I got it all free, my younger siblings where so great full to wake up to a warm house and a warm meal all prepared for them again, I got a job at a bakery, graveyard shift making Syrian flat bread, and it seemed like it would be ok to start but it wasn't, I started to have mother issues, After working all night and getting everyone out in the morning, I wanted to get to bed, but was not allowed to, my mother said I don't care what hours you work, no one sleeps in the day time around here. Get out of bed, she would grab my feet and pull me out of bed, why? I just worked all night, I was giving her money doing chores helping "everyone", just like I said I would, I even got food stamps and I gave her all of them, for the first time in months they had a refrigerator full of food, but I was not allowed to sleep in day time, she even would poke me with the end of a broom handle if I fell asleep, it hurt, I ended up going out into the woods to sleep, sometimes the car, Why did she do this to me? I needed to sleep. I worked 11:00 PM till 6:00 AM, It got better when I got a job in the day time working on cars. And I would soon meet a woman that I would marry, I spent little time at home I stayed in motels, I began to really dislike my mother again, and why was she so hostile, and so very controlling? It was her way or the high way? She was always right, never wrong about anything, she picked my sisters boyfriends and my girlfriends, if she didn't like you,

you had it, You were made miserable, with her endless complaining, and I looked at my poor dad drunk dying in the corner, There was no love there, no care, as a child many times I came home in the evening to find my mother with her head flat down on the kitchen table stoned drunk. Always saying she was waiting for dad to fall asleep, she didn't want to go up there and be with him, all she got out of it was a baby, so! I guess my dad was no great lover. Or it was my mother's fault the way she was brought up by her strict catholic mother, she always told us because her dad was sick in the hospital so long, she raised her brothers while her mother worked, and was treated as a servant more like the help, she was never allowed to sit in their chairs at the table, she had her own spot and would have to clean up after everyone after dinner, and get her brothers ready for school, Men in the household where kings, like she always told me "I" would be, but I feel it was not so true, I feel she resented the treatment she got, and as much as she wanted that boy (me) her son the one she always dreamed of having. Only brought to surface her anger, the anger she had for having to do all that work as a child, And to become like a mother so young and in the end get so little respect from her brothers, In my life knowing her brothers I could see how they thought so much better of themselves, and so little of her, So much they competed between themselves, who would do better, who would make the most, in the end who would retire with it all, and to them my dad was just a blue collar worker, he wore a uniform, that meant he was a lowly working nobody to them and they had no respect for him, she also meant little to them, just there maid sister, They thought of woman's as servants each wanted an Asian wife so they would get waited on hand and foot, one of her brothers did marry one but she was a feisty one, she had him wrapped around her finger.

I swear they would have ordered one through the mail but my grandmother would not allow that, It was always as if it was my mom's lucky day if she got a visit from one of them, I always felt my mother actually resented me as a boy, I brought back those feelings of her she had as a child, having me was not what she expected, or was not what she really wanted, it was only a belief installed in her, in her upbringing, that a son was so important, and it had to be me, me! the son that wasn't, I had got back to my friend I knew from high school, who was a super good mechanic, His brother too and we would reconnect, grow into a great friendship, I got a job working on cars putting alarms, stereos, all custom dash board accessories factory and after market and would soon learn factory and aftermarket air conditioning installation, the three of us would go out on weekends and days off to do side jobs, I learned all around mechanic work, And was soon out doing my own work part time after work. I had learned a lot from these two boys, there dad was a mechanic at New England drag way, and a Tool and Die maker, but what a temper, something I would find in that trade myself, the men it are stressed out all day long in a state of sever concentration all your senses, feel, touch, smell sight, sound, are all pushed to their maximum limits as you build out your die, they knew all kinds of tune up tricks to really get a car flying, no one in the area had a faster street car than these two, none, And they were sleepers, junk boxes all cut out inside to make them light, no nice paint, no upholstery just seats, old GTO's and Pontiac tempests, and Catalina's they just blew the doors off cars that kids dumped thousands into and left them way back in the dust. Just embarrassed them, Bill would become my closet friend in those years and would be the best man at my wedding, And I would hear rumors he was gay, but I never asked and he never told me, once when I cross dressed and I just changed, he came over to visit, we shared a joint, I looked at the end after a couple hit's it had lipstick on it, and he noticed to. but never said anything, I would have told him if I had gotten the chance, Only several years later I would be his pall bearer at his funeral, he would be killed in an auto mobile accident in 1985, right now It was July 1976 and someone got a pile of Elton John tickets for the July 3rd concert and I grabbed one I think it was a friends brother, it was to be quite a concert planned in Foxboro, Elton John came down out of a helicopter playing a piano and was dropped on the stage, And it got better from there, what a showman, I had never really liked much of his music, but up on stage with that band he had, he was amazing, I was smoking pot with everyone and dropped acid, the whole experience was just full of excitement. I was in one of my happier moods in a while, it had been so long since I got away from feeling so depressed and let go of my struggles, and I look down to where all my friends are I see a girl sitting alone, but sometimes bill comes up and talks to her but leaves for long periods of time, I start to wonder if there together, I watch, and nothing, bill is making no moves, just small talk. It doesn't appear they are together, a half hour goes buy and still no closeness, Bill is further away and not really paying attention to her, the night is so wonderful, it's almost midnight, the concert will be over once they light off the fireworks at the end of the concert on the fourth, It will be July 4th 1976 and the firework display planned was going to be real big. And one thing is missing right now that will make it all perfect, my arms around someone, someone to hug and hold onto at the end of the concert when the fireworks went off, and so I went, where I got the courage I don't know, it just seemed I had to do it, I sat beside her and said hello enjoying the concert? And she said yes, and we introduced each other, I asked, are you with anyone here? She said no. I came alone just with my sister and some friends, we both giggle admitting we are both tripping away And having a great time, and I reach over and put my arm around her waist and pull her in tight, looking for a reaction, I see a smile on her face, and then I hear I loud explosion, the fireworks where going off, and what a firework display, It went on at least half hour nonstop all the big stuff like a grand finally all in one, It was now the fourth of July we sometimes disagree over the date we met she says the 3rd I say the 4th to this day, But I know when I approached her it was close enough to the fourth, At midnight, and the bad part was when we left she asked I rode home with her so I said ok and waved good bye to my friends I came with, only to find her car was towed, and we had to walk two hours to find it, we would see each other at a few more concerts and have a few dates, some not so good, she drank heavy and was flirty with guys sitting in the seats, even get a beer off one while I sat there watching, it felt very humiliating to me and I confronted her about it, I did not like that at all, she was with me, if she wanted beer from another guy then I told her to stay with him, I will go find someone else to be with, she also almost got beat up in the girls line going into the bathroom's, She would try cutting in line drunk out of her mind, and there was no way I could pull ten girls off her, I stood waiting for a cat fight like everyone else, woman take 4 times longer to pee, why they have the same amount of restrooms in a building is beyond me, guys!, in and out!, Woman, they take forever, and it's not their fault, later as a woman myself I would really miss that standing up to pee, when you are really in a hurry what a giveaway that was, and men they just think woman are in there looking in the mirror all that time, Oh no! wrong, it takes longer to pee as a woman, woman need more and bigger rest rooms, at least three for every men's room, I really did not think our relationship would work out, plus I had my gender issue still, and to me it bothered and depressed me daily. I wasn't thinking a relationship was not going to be good for me at all right now. I had something to find out about myself first, I did not want to hurt anyone, fall in love and get hurt, or hurt who I got involved with, I was afraid to let myself go, my soul was locked inside surrounded by a cold breeze and an empty feeling, the only feeling I could fill myself now with was sadness and grief, it was a strong feeling. It filled the emptiness I had, and always, that depression has a way of wrapping around you like a warm blanket fooling your soul into thinking it has brought you to a safe warm place where you soon may end your life, plans of suicide become long fantasy's long daydreams that carry me away for days, as I plan, and grieve and cry, and there is a feeling you get when you try to snap yourself out of it, an empty cold chill hangs on the outer edges of your skin, and I would remember being in love, being with my soul mate, the one I lost and it was so painful The feeling of being cut in two is powerful, I had seen her around and had heard she was with someone now, I had no desire to go into her life and try to take away anything that was making her happy, I hoped she was well and in love, and was having all the happiness she wanted, and I in no way even wanted to interrupt it in any way, I only at that time in my life hoped I would fall In love again myself somehow, it had to be there somewhere, but I knew there was a part of me that had to learn to love myself first, before I could love anyone or anything, there was me, I was learning you really have to love yourself before you can love others, or it's not as real. Or you will make mistakes and only bring pain to both, I knew I was a woman in a man's body and who I was became stronger with age, and not going away. This new woman I met came by to visit one day, we had to talk about our new relationship, it was not taking off well, And I felt my mother resented me being with someone, she wanted all my attention now, My dad was closing in on death he had almost 7-8 months left in his life, So together she and I went off to a nice secluded spot I had for myself in the woods near my home, A mossy little hill, it was like nature threw out a warm soft carpet to sit or lie down on. And I explained to her then all my feelings, about my gender and my identity issues, and how I have struggled my entire life, and also had never gotten over my first love, and felt that my gender issue was a big part of her leaving me, I had frightened someone I loved away and was afraid it would always happen to me, and having a relationship with me was not a good idea,

If she really ever knew me I would scare her away, I would not blame her for not seeing me again, this was hard she knew all my friends, was she going to tell everyone about this? all my friends were going to find out and walk away, I may have been about to lose everything in my life I had, and have to start all over, even move away somewhere. All this went through my mind, as we sat there, she said little, she asked, you are telling me you really feel like you are a woman? Just born in a man's body? that's sounds hard to even think of never mind believe, and she asked me do I wear woman's cloths a lot, I said I never really have any or the time and privacy, so no not really, it's just a problem in my mind I need to solve, and soon we left, with just a smile on her face she drove away, I didn't see her for a while I did not think she would be back, but a few weeks later she came by and said want to hang out? she had a six pack of beer, and said every things ok, let's Just go talk, and we went out for a drive, my mother was pissed, I was never home much now, I either slept in the car all night or we pooled our paychecks that week and stayed in motel rooms whenever possible, and a few times she even let me cross dress for a while, she wanted to see this side of me, one night she pulled a dress out of her pocket book and brought all her makeup, and said she wanted to see what I looked like and I did not mind, I thought she liked me at first, and I was hoping she would like this side of me always, there was no room for me at the house, less I wanted to throw a sleeping bag down on the floor by the fireplace, I had no bedroom or privacy there, what was I to do.? But it seemed to anger my mother, she didn't like someone else with me, and barely spoke to either of us when we visited, In February she comes to me and tells me, she may be pregnant, I was at first surprised, it was so real, it was like the party is over, wake up, The world just shook me out of bed and threw me into the cold, and said you have to take care of another human being besides yourself, another part of "you", your own, a baby, and it hit me! A baby! I was having a baby, how cool was that, I dreamed of having one, only it was myself that wanted to carry, I had all my life this overwhelming feeling this very strong desire to have a baby grow inside me, as if I needed it, I was so sad I could never in my life feel a life growing inside me, also it reminds me of my aunt when I was told she could not have babies, she or my uncle had something wrong with them, and being pregnant it would be another connection to my soul I so much needed to warm, comfort. and help make it feel it was not alone, and also when my wife was pregnant it was the only time in my life I experienced the feeling of jealousy, never with other woman that would be taken away from me, I expected and accepted it as part of my life, and I just let go, but when my wife carried, I felt it I was really wanting to be her, I pray god's forgiveness for my mixed feelings daily and hope that if I am to be forgiving when my time here ends, that I may enter the home of his heaven and into the arms of his mother Mary, and the mother of Jesus herself will accept me in, and as a woman, and also that I may be a soul so happy! that I may be allowed to enter heaven with a tear, I tell her not to worry we will be ok, our love will grow along with our family and we will be fine, I was not in love but I hoped that if she loved me and took in the part of me that was my soul and I felt she loved that side of me, I hoped for a chance, again that there may be a time I fall in love again. And We move into a small two bedroom apt. with her sister and her sister's boyfriend, But after a couple months we feel not so wanted there we have problems with them and decide to go off on our own, Right at this time, my dad dies, My wife breaks the news to me after work, I hadn't yet told him he was to be a grandfather, he lay dying in a hospital bed and I was coming in soon to tell him, I thought that telling him his first son, was having a baby would help, maybe give him some strength. But I never got the chance, he was gone, two weeks after he died I had a nightmare that we had my father in a sheet, "all of us", the entire family, carrying him to his grave like we had him in a sack. He was wrapped in a sheet, except for his face, I looked down at him and he opened one eye and looked at me. Just as his body hovered above the hole in the ground we were just about to drop him in, and then we all just let go, and walked away wiping the dirt off our hands, I woke up shaking, it seemed so real, I had a guilty feeling I may have had something to do with my father drinking more at the end and giving up, my mom kept teasing about his girlfriend, he may have had a mistress and my mother did not seem to mind, I didn't know what type of relationship it was or even if it was real. Just that she teased they met at a bar occasionally, and my mom was glad it was the other woman and not her, I never took it seriously, then one night the phone rings, I was visiting my parents it's her, and she thinks I am my dad, we sound alike, she wants to go out, I didn't know what to say I was caught off guard, I just said I can't get out at the moment, And she seemed really upset, and argued about it for a few minutes wanting me to explain myself, and all I could say was I just can't make it out tonight. I looked up at my dad, I wanted to get him and try to get his attention but he was watching television and already drinking as usual, but I was a astonished and taken a little off my feet at the moment, Finding out my dad really had a mistress, and what to say next before she got mad and hung up, which she did, real loud, I heard she never called back, I noticed my dad get sadder and more withdrawn always looking at his watch. And I noticed my mom saying how come your girlfriend doesn't call anymore? Did I just ruin what little bit of love left in my dad's life unknowingly? I still feel bad afterwards to this day, I should have gotten him but she thought I was him so fast and it all happened so fast, I try hard not to blame myself, the saddest part about my dad dying was Christmas morning he got all his strength he had left to get up and watch us open our Christmas presents, and soon he just collapsed right there in front of us all, and we got an ambulance, he never came back home again, Christmas day was our last day at home with our father, And I was no stranger to depression and being alone, and soon would even shut myself out and go twenty years into celibacy because I got to hurt and pulled away, Every day is a day of thinking of a way to end my life without a lot of pain, my father did it slowly and painfully. And it was always her in my death fantasy. I was always a woman in my coffin or a woman hanging by her neck on a rope, and yet my worst fear of dying was the people around me would dress me as a man in my coffin and hide who I was, and I would never rest in peace, what horrible thoughts to have all this time, seemed like forever they were there, I would walk hand in hand through life with depression and the thoughts of suicide daily, not a day would go by ever without one thought or fantasy of it, not ever, there is no feeling of belonging anywhere, It's like the world is a party you weren't invited to but went anyway, Most people want you to just leave, some will talk but not really be to friendly, you will find some very close friends but they are all under pressure to reject you from somewhere, you feel it all around, It's as scary as being a child lost in a big department store, lost in a sea of unfamiliar faces, The only friendly ones are the ones at the reception desk comforting you while you wait for someone who loves you, to come and find you.

You walk out the door every day in a battle of your own will to keep surviving. And hope someday for an answer or an end to all of this. And the one thing you would love is one friend to say it's ok, don't worry, I am here for you, you are not all alone, if those words are like food and you are starving for them, so bad, that if you got a taste you may bite your tongue or your own finger, And all of this just has to be kept inside no one knows but you, and what you are going through and feeling, I would soon get the biggest rejection in my life soon, and from my own mother, for a stranger, we I moved to an apartment in Quincy Ma a call came, again my wife again has news of a death, it's my uncle, my mother's oldest brother, he has just had a massive heart attack and died, I have gone to see my grandmother, the house in a state of weeping, my grandmother and my mother were in shock even my grandfather, Who never got along with his son well was in state of disbelief, This would be a terrible loss, He was all my mother really had, except another brother she barely ever saw, a younger brother who lived most of his life in the west coast, the one that just died was going to retire soon and stay with his sister and help her fix up her home and keep her there in a nicer rebuilt home, I was getting along with him for the first time ever in my life, my wife and I met him out walking with our first baby, we were not married yet but he still called her my wife, he showed he respected her, He was riding his bicycle in the park bare cove Hingham, where we ourselves always walked, He was making blue bird nests and putting them in the park in the exact places, to attract the bird, so the blue bird would return, he said it was almost eradicated because it will attack you, but only if it thinks you are too close to it eggs or babies, and not really the aggressive bird people claimed, and he wanted to bring the species back to this area, he would stop and talk to us, I felt his genuine friendship for the first time in my life, we never really had in the past, he was more fond of my sisters and took them everywhere, I was always left out, If I did get to go I was neglected, I was lucky to find water, if we got any breakfast at a table he bought me a bowl of oatmeal, and my sisters got piles of pancakes and bacon, and deserts, always treated me as if he just didn't want me there, he would even try to gyp me when I cut his lawn for him, he would try to forget and take off without paying me, many times my grandmother paid me, and said damn thing what a cheapskate but he mellowed with age and he had even smoked marijuana with the artist friend of ours, I was very sad he had died, I was really just getting to know him and I had all my life wanted to, he was very intelligent and was telling me things about black holes in outer space before any of it ever came out public, now his brother would come and change everything, He would take so much of what his brother had, for himself! He did not leave his sister much to build with, He and his wife Considered her(my mother) and all of us, nothing but peasants, and we deserved nothing better than to always be the beggars they called us, and they took everything my uncle had and left claiming there was nothing there but later would own a multimillion dollar mansion in one of California's richest counties, my uncles aunt hung out with the actors on the sitcom, (house wives) And my mother had no back bone to get a lawyer and audit his sudden wealth, he left his only sister to die in the end penniless, and he goes to church every Sunday, but that wasn't the worst of it, My sister the 4th child, the one behind me, brings home a new boyfriend, she met him buying a car, He was the salesman selling her the car, which she had ordered special, took forever to get and came in the wrong color in the end, and was the wrong model, what she ordered never came, It was probably never ordered. he waited for one to come in that would match as close as possible and hope that after waiting months to get it, she would take anything that was close enough, and she did, all of a sudden he moved in and is making all the decisions for my mother, and driving my sisters car like it was his own, and my mother she is hypnotized by this man, He has her convinced that she should sell her home and go to cape cod, buy land near the ocean and he was a carpenter he would build homes for her all along the beaches of the cape, she would be rich, I tell her to stay where she is, at least wait two or three years the value of her home is going to shoot way up, or if she sells it to let me buy it, but everything she replied back to me was I will ask him, He is so wonderful and he knows everything, I would tell her you don't really know him he could be conning you, don't sell it, she would just get angry and say I'll tell him just what you said to me! you'll see what he can do, he's wonderful, he can do anything, you'll see, soon her home is on the market and it very pricey for me, so I talk to some banks and find out how easy it is to buy a house that has been passed down through the family like this, And being it was my fathers, fathers home then going to me, all I had to do was sign and move in, as long as the value was what my mom would take, I could buy it my credit was very good and getting the mortgage was no issue for me, I called, I was hoping to buy it, she said I have good news I have sold the house, at first I was ok with it, I thought she got the very high price she was asking, but she didn't, she got one third of it and after taxes and repairs they made her do, about 1/5 of what she should have gotten from me, I was horrified, and she did it all behind my back with this boyfriend of my sister, never told me about dropping the price, They just sold it and tried to sneak off, without saying a word, I just couldn't believe this, all my life being told that I was her "son", that one she would need, especially when the day came and if dad died, and he did, her closet brother too, she said how much she would need me! And when the time really comes she goes to a stranger, a drunken car salesman. Who in three years takes every penny she has, And flushes everything the family has or could ever have had right down the toilet, He was dead in about ten years from alcohol poisoning leaving behind 3 children and my sister, The house they had bought down in the cape, with the money from two homes in Hingham, became uninhabitable and was condemned, for a while my mother was away with another sister the kids there partied and smashed the home to pieces, and it was torn down, everything he built fell down, he had lied, he never built anything in his entire life, and before he died the police were looking for a man who was going to old woman and saying he would do repairs, take a big deposit of $1,500 or more and never return, it was him, and the funny thing is he worked as a security guard in a hospital, and new every cop in town and even had a gun, He would sit out in his car and eat a whole bucket of Kentucky fried chicken with a bottle of vodka while inside his kids were waiting for dinner, my sister would find him in the morning on her way to work, passed out with chicken bones all over him, he was almost a police officer, but was drunk all the time, they fired him, I didn't speak to my mother for almost ten years except for a few visits when she had asked for help, and I wondered why, this guy was supposed to be so wonderful, I would get there and find him leaning against a wall using it to hold himself up. His pants soaked in urine and a bottle of vodka in his hand, claiming he was not drinking, and had not touched a drop of liquor all day, My grandmother before she died asked me what I thought of my Mothers new home, I said I was horrified and was totally disgusted with what she got for what she had, she made a big mistake, she bought a dump a half-finished house, and the seller lied about the size of the lot, two years after she moved in someone built a home on land she thought was hers, right in her back yard, I wish I was there the day she realized she screwed up and lost her son and seen the expression on her face, when she realized this guy was a bum, and took her for everything she had, it must have been very close to the look I got the very first time she saw me dressed as a woman, i it just made me snap I just lost it, I was not her son, all that weight lifted off me. It felt like a relief. I felt like if I had become a woman, if I had found a way now, what difference would it make to my mother? If I told her it made it so much easier now. In fact I looked forward to it, where before I dreaded it, I was never the son she wanted, it was all a lie, a big myth, Her feelings towards me as a son from that point meant nothing to me anymore, she threw me out for a stranger, she took away the family's home, My Fathers. Fathers, families home, it was all our home, It's what we all called it "home," without any regards at all to anyone, and it also angered my father's side of the family, that she gave none of them a chance to buy it.

There was a land dispute they believed half was there's and if I bought it I would have divided it for them and kept the peace in the family, they all came from Prince Edwards Island. My father's mother and brother both had a deed for the land but my grandmother beat her brother to have it notarized making it legally hers, they bought it from a senile old man who sold it to both of them, and there was plenty to share my grandmothers brother had a small house on the corner lot but only on a very small lot, and I could not believe she just took off and tried to sneak away, they never spoke to her again for that, she lost most of her family for this man, we have to aunts in Arlington we visited almost every holiday and slept over many long weekends, our closest of friends, they even warned my mother and she told them off, They never spoke again for about 15 years, but very little when they did. People that once hugged and loved each other now just stood there and just said hi, we lost a great relationship, it took years before they saw us again, I always wondered who he really married, my mother or my sister, I could not wait for the day to come if ever. And I would tell her finally I am your daughter not your son anymore, I did I get that day, I told her on the phone, All I remember is, It got real quiet after I told her, she was shocked, and I said I always thought you knew, but she denied it, I said what about that doctor you took me into in Boston he asked me, I thought you put him up to it, but she said no, she remembered the appointment though, My youngest sister told me later I nearly killed her from the shock, and why did I even tell her?

I told her I felt she always knew and kept it from me, it was no real surprise to her, otherwise I would not have, but I think it was the reality when I finally came out and finally said it! In the back of her mind she thought I might come out and say it someday, and I finally did and it hit her hard all these years waiting for it, and it came, the first time she saw me dressed as a woman she did not recongnice me at all. One of her own children and she could not see the old me, I felt so good to finally tell her without guilt attached to it, but right now at this moment in time with the kids and family I was a real man now, making money working as a tool and die maker, a black belt in karate, working on automobiles on the side had several daughters, always had money in my pocket, grew a beard, I hated it felt like someone pulled me by the chin all day, but it looked good on me, it was the best look I had as a man ever, I could have been a double for Paul McCartney when he had his, And was told that by many people, I wore leather vests, walked around with an angry and stressed out look all the time, some people asked why is your fist so tight? you look like you want to hit someone or start a fight, I put all my feelings deep inside and went along with my life, I hadn't cross dressed much in over ten years, I really ever get too much, I felt that my wife did not really accept that part of me, like I had hoped, I believed if she paid just a little more attention to that side of me. And took the time to be patient and nurture my most important and wonderful part of me. while we were still very young and growing she may well have had a wonderful husband, and lover But many times she would say I don't want to be with her today, and it was not like I did it daily or every weekend, or monthly, It would be six months or more that I would get a day for myself to dress nice, Sometimes I asked and sometimes I did not, either way I always got rejected, and that side of me just pulled back inside, it was hurt, she did not take the time to get to know that side of me at all and to me it was important, I needed to nurture that side of me not lock it away, it was the better side of me, my spirit and soul, she wanted me to keep it a secret which is okay but if I dress why get upset when no one is here? and I am not looking for it as a sexual routine, I just wanted her to know "her", "me" Anytime that we did have sex she coaxed me into it more than it was me, It was still a little awkward to feel like a man with woman's clothes on having sex but it was as close and I can get. and in the right time and place and if she knows the right things to say she can bring me in close enough to feel both our hearts, but if she if she rejects me in any way and I feel that side of me is not wanted it will close up, and go away, I will draw my soul in and keep it inside to protect it from being hurt, just a few times when we lived in our second Quincy apt, A few other times in the other apartment we lived a short time in Quincy, On a day off and no one was home, or the motels we stayed in but still just those were quick peeks that's all. And when you have sex all you clothes come off anyway, I still never really had a day yet to just sit and relax and be me, and I am already 23 years old. Our first baby was in the crib It was thanksgiving, although my wife had always seen a little about what I look like but not really so much what I would act like or act out, I was so busy working I never really had a day to really just take and have as a day dressed as a woman so she planned a nice thanksgiving dinner at home, and bought me a nice little surprise, A nice beige lacey dress for dinner Over that year I had saved things for myself in a little corner of a draw, makeup foundations and, lipsticks, stockings, Eyeliners, corsets, garters, never wore or used them much just storing them, I felt like I was putting pieces of myself together, and storing a little treasures, and although it all stayed in a draw most of the time, it felt like it was "mine" and a little bit of me, not really me, but so far the closet I ever got, like I was starting to build a person, together that thanksgiving, we both cooked and prepared dinner got dressed, she helped me with my makeup and anything else I needed I did not really know much about makeup just from watching and reading, I never had a lot of practice to really do a professional job, But she has learned things all her life and is very helpful with hints and ways to use it, It shocked her at first that I had taken the extra effort to shave my legs, but! it was what I wanted, It was amazing to see myself standing there again in a mirror, and this is the first time, there is no fear of someone looking in, or finding me, catching me being "bad" or weak, I did not have to hide. I could really just relax and enjoy this and feel what I was missing. And I just feel right, that warm feeling that just warms my soul comes out of me, the chill fades. I feel right, I can't explain it but I feel like I am supposed too. I see a person I want to be forever, and share with everyone. with her appearance all these softer emotions just pour into me, like software being downloaded in a computer, I am much kinder, gentler, And we have an for myself an unforgettable dinner and night, ` My first time having sex dressed as a woman, In nice stockings, garters and corsets, and nice polished nails I did not expect it to be as gentle and as sincere as it was, I hoped maybe we would again but she always needs to coax me into this. I am a little shy about it, but I also like being coaxed, it's like a courting feel, I let her have a little bit of domination over me she is wanting me, and I am so willingly surrendering, like a woman I like to be hit on and in the darkness of the room after penetration, I can't tell who is who. I can imagine I am in a females body, for the first time, I can really imagine I am a woman, Along with all the lingerie the smell of the perfumes the silkiness of the stockings and the stickiness of lipsticks, The pull of the garter straps and soft human skin, and the kinder gentler touch I have, all these things together bring out strong feminine feelings that I just want to always have and I just want to let go, and she is saying the right things to me, the things a woman likes to hear, how soft my lips are and my "gentle touch", my loving way to hug and hold her. And although not a woman, this is as close to it at the time I get, Finally someone likes to be treated gently, all those nice little things add something more to it, and her gentle touch back, all just fill me with a feeling of life I never experienced before, and the gentleness of love that goes with all this is more than any I thought I ever would create with the touch of my own hands, As if I touched with my soul and not my body, I had become like an angel of touch and pleasure, and hoped that this would never end, but it does, a few times my wife is out, I am just dressed sitting watching television waiting for her to come home and just talk not jump into the bedroom just sit and talk, and she is disappointed I am dressed, she says I don't want to be with her tonight, I am so confused, and hurt, I thought her was me, I did not want to separate myself into two people like that, If she wanted to add this as a sexual fantasy and just use me as a sex toy, Whenever she was in the mood and add this to our routines I wanted no part of it, I would not like it, I went into this relationship honestly and told her all my feelings, when you tell someone you feel like you are a woman born in a man's body you cannot explain it any more clear, as much as it was for even myself to understand what I was going through, that is a good explanation, and also I fully understood it was just the same for her as anyone else, I would tell, I to this day cannot figure out why she still stays here with me and be so unhappy, now that she has really realized she married a woman, and as for the sex part of it if it became just a routine like that, I would soon have that boy in a dress feeling I do not want at all, It would bring back the feeling when I was a very young boy and when I wore a dress and masturbated the very first time and how awkward a feeling it was, to look like a girl doing what a boy does, It just feels wrong, looks wrong and is very uncomfortable, and does not work, I get nowhere with it, masturbation for me was a horrible part of my life, I hated, it was a need, more than anything else, like going to the bathroom to pee, it was something that built up inside you, It grew into multiple cells and became over loaded as you waited in long time between encounters, or breaking down and do your best to remove your inhibitions and stop the pain, A lot of pain, frustration, and being hard on yourself to the point you can no longer even walk is not a good idea but if you are inhibited like me. you may have some bad days, Ejaculation is painful, there is no pleasure to it at all, just pain, a solution for me when I was young was to use a woman's menstrual cycle, monthly", 3-5 times in one month, It was the only way I could even deal with it emotionally, I even put a little check on the 28th day on calenders so I could know, and allow myself to even touch myself that way, one of the reasons I would also soon hate my penis so much, I did not want to deal with it at all, I wanted to do was just cut it off me, I kept my Grand Fathers old straight razor for many, many years after I moved away and kept it of only using it for that one purpose, it was very sharp and I took the belt to sharpen it with, It became like a padlock on a prison door It had to come off and I did not want to be a man dressed as a woman just for sex either, it was not going to feel right, my brain knows what my body is doing especially if it's routine I will not fool myself, and end up sick and depressed for days, weeks, months and I get nauseous and depressed and often suicidal, just for that, a few moments, it's not worth it, I just wait it out till I get over it, I have 3-5 days in pain so bad going up and down stairs is not a good idea, and cramps in my, stomach, you can do it! you can live without it, you just have to be patient, it will go away, you can live without sex although I do not recommend it at all when you get older you become more afraid of it, I have not even kissed a woman on the lips in over twenty years as I write this book, I am like a virgin again, I am so scared I will even kiss wrong, Or touch to gentle and scare her away, But if you are young, get help early don't put yourself through all this pain don't try to put it away and be a man, Get help early if you need to change, do it young and have a natural sex life, don't punish yourself, like I did, It hurts real bad emotionally in the end,

I have become so frightened of an encounter, one mistake and I get a rejection and I most likely will kill myself, as quick as that, and warn no one, and if I am with someone who knows this and they reject me, in the end and know what I might do, I will not even tell them, it won't come out of me, my planning has begun, I will just go do it. You lose a lot more than you will ever know in the end, If you hold back and try to go it alone and try to be the man you are not, I put my things back in my draw and there they will stay for many, many months and years at a time, I went to work in a factory, just pulling handles, I worked hard showed up every day did my share or more, helped others, I loved it the days flew by. I got over time a lot, and soon got a job running a larger manual turret lathe, was taught by a woman to run it, she had been there since world war II when woman ran the factories, I had met several older woman that where tool and die makers there, when they were younger, I just did the same as they told me, I worked hard got everything done. No complaints or rejected parts, and was giving another chance to become a tool and die maker, what a trade, a real man's trade, macho all the way, a room full of genius want to bee's and half really were the other half thought they were, And the competition was like sports. Someone had to be the super home run hitter, god help you if you screwed up. Men gossip real bad, especially when they got you in a weak moment, and you made a mistake, It was written down and used against you years later, damage to any tool or die running in a press at high speed would or could cost tens to hundreds of thousands to repair, "If the press or a person was hurt, even the risks of you almost screwing up was going to get you an ass chewing And a feeling of letting you know how small you really are, and accidents are all over. I saw a lot of operators lose hands and fingers; some dies had to have a special pressure plate set with the stroke of the press so you could not stick the tips of your fingers in them. to chop off the tops of them to collect insurance, some operators made money on their fingers on purpose, The work itself is very technical working to .00010 to an inch with hardened steels and tonnage of impact up to 300 tons easy, At 250 strokes or more a minute when the boss was asked to send his best man on a particular job and he sent you, It was a good feeling, Pay meant little when you felt good about what you did, you where the man, coming to fix tools no one else could and get a group of 30 or more people back in there place working and producing and making money for your company, The presidents, of multi, multimillion dollar companies new me by my first name and visited my work bench, looked at all the pictures of my family and knew them all by name. I was somebody, and I was fast, lighting speed, my martial arts training was up to 4-6 hours a day in between work and play, I was so fast and powerful with a punch. I could knock someone twice my size off their feet with one punch! flat on their back, if I hit someone real hard in the head there brain would explode, I was lethal, I was working a real man's trade, I met with other martial artists training like myself behind buildings and practiced for real, we beat on each other till we got exhausted, all my feelings about that female identity had been quietly pushed away, but still there for those days I needed comfort, or the stress was too much Being what I wasn't and being this good at it meant a lot of work, physical and mental, That little box! My secret jewelry box! She would sometimes just appear in my mind out of nowhere, a candle was lit there burning for her, one I had lit so long ago, now lit up to keep her warm, standing there with her hands folded in front down at her sides, just looking up. And wondering where we were, in a nice dress that lit up in the candle's warm amber light, I would put her away like a treasure, I knew she was a part of my identity and that little box was always my safe place to go, though I would become a successful male, and a very good dad. My children never went to bed hungry, I had as a child, and I knew how it hurt my father more than it hurt us he could not feed us that night, we made the best of it, my mother would by cake and ice cream so we would feel happy, I know as bad as our relationship was I am sure on those nights he could not provide for us he must have cried, I know I sure would have, and the big old house was way too much for him alone to care for, just to heat it was a strain, I was always cold, I never had a warm home till I got my first apt, and as I cared for my own children. I would have many days of a lot of sadness, loneliness disappointments, doubts and make mistakes, have worries and concerns as anyone else would, maybe more or less but I had to do my best to be like a man and keep it all in, like it does not bother me, and because that is what a man does, I had no way to let it out, but I had found a way in, and it was into my little box I would go and travel as her, but I could only stay for short times and would come to that box when I was really troubled and scared, and also you know and learn what most of men are really like, and you will find that many are not too good, And things they say and do to woman and want to do to someone like you are things that if you are old and have been without a male partner like myself and have only been with woman, than I would think most likely like myself you yourself would stay with a woman, But if you where to get help early in your life it would be different the life you would have would be of a normal female and your choice of a mate would start off naturally, and it would be a moment to take your time with your choices and not rush into them, I hope when you are done reading I can help you make a choice, Being with them to much you know what all there weakness and faults are and I was there, I did it, I made it, I should be ok, But I have learned to much about the darker side of the male ego, and I wish I hadn't, although I have met a few good ones, they are out there, you need to be a strong patient woman like the rest of them looking for that Mr. Right, I know now why I hear woman say that, and I would do cross dressers an injustice, they treat woman like gods, And now my grandmother has died, and my mother was now just about penniless again, about to lose everything she has, she is raising my sisters kids while my fourth sister also works, My mother ends up having to go back to work herself, supposedly her golden retirement years working in a candy store just so she can eat, I asked her about my grandmother's house and that she promised me I could have her half when it's sold because she sold my dad's home and this was a way to pay back what she had done, but when I asked, she told me my sister's husband needed every penny she could get to finish her home in the cape, And could not let me have her half, and I could not buy that one either, Not with the steep price her younger brother put on it.

And I loved that house and the time I lived there and went to high school although I was in such a troubled time of my life, I loved my grandparents so much, and they were being erased from my memories, because of a stranger who walked into our lives and said he would make it all a wonderful life for us all, Just like a near death experience my memories all flooded me and I just break down, I hadn't cried in a long time, tears again, where have they been? I feel something poor into my body, And it's heavy as it rises like warm oils slowly filling inside of my entire body, making me warm and heavy, every part of me is in grief and getting warm and flushed, as it comes up from the bottom to were my eyes await at the edge and for a few moments lingers at the cusp of the wave before it comes out in the relief of tears, waiting to die bringing out all your pain, tears are like medicine, they bring out of your body all the things that come into your life and try to bring pain deep into your soul, and they take that pain and sacrifice themselves for you, as they leap to their death at the outer edge of where you see the world from, so you can heal, And I cannot control it, and I do not really want too, I need too, it is my time to let my soul heal, I know why I am crying, I have been betrayed by my mother, and my wife has no real feelings for "me" the true "me", Alone at the house, I am going to see her again, I got out my clothes makeup everything I needed, locked my door, I had one of those very rare opportunity's that I was alone that day at least a couple hours, And soon I felt it was if I put away and hid an old friend that I was embarrassed and ashamed of, I looked at her and just saw how right I looked and felt again, I was warm again inside of my soul. And my heart, I had decided it was time to find help again, time to look for answers, look for doctors again, it's been so many years now I am about 33 years old, there must be doctors now, I got every phone book, finally almost a twenty year search may have finally produced a result, So I make an appointment, My first meeting I get right to the point, it is the first thing I say to him, To explain myself, I looked at everyone, every doctor, every field, anything, It took another two years. And during that time I did not cross dress, but for only a few moments at a time, just to get my peek, a look at what and who I hoped will be coming, there was too much stress at home and work, to really find time to relax and enjoy a few hours, I waited for every new phone book like a kid waiting for a toy ordered from a catalogue, and I find my first in Brookline ma, a sex therapist! all types gay straight marital, "gender disorders, finally there is that word "gender" and I go in and see him and Just like I did when I was 16 years old at a clinic in Quincy and got thrown out three sessions late, I tell him I feel like I was born a woman, in a man's body, and his reaction and question back is very unexpected, he pauses and looks at me for about one minute, he asks when you dress as a woman do you masturbate, I said no! He said no? Right I said no, no again? He asked! That's unusual! I said why? I said I find that very uncomfortable, he said, you're not a transsexual then! No way, you cannot be one, I said why? He said they all do! Every transsexual will cross dress then masturbate, it's what they do, it's part of their makeup, it's a need they have. And it's how they fantasy themselves as woman! And are having intercourse, Oh! I see, but I explained I can't concentrate fully on my feelings as a woman if I am aroused with an erection, I like to experience that when I am dressed, and want to explore my female side emotionally I do not want to use it as a fetish and just like sex and like all men when you are done you want to leave, it would be over, You would want to take all your woman's clothes off, it seems like too much work, and I told him. I also feel like the act of masturbation for me while I have a penis, is a boys thing, and I feel like a boy when I do that, and very awkward in a dress I get an almost out of body feeling, I do not like it, they are what I find out later are called panic attacks, and I do not want to masturbate in woman's clothes it's very wrong, I said when I was very young about six years old I get that out of body feeling at school when I would look over at all the girls, when they separated us boy girl boy girl, and then I told him if I have to relieve myself I would rather get that part over with first then enjoy myself dressed as a woman without any distraction, especially an erection, it would just depress me, I feel backwards. he said then I will work on making you happy as a man and we will work on the woman part later, I was not happy with that, I did not see him after that but I got the number and name of his associate it was on his business card, That masturbation issue would be an issue with doctors I seek, and in books I would read on the subject, so I have to answer it honestly in this book, let me say that when I am alone by myself for that purpose, it's strange, it's a boy thing, the whole movement, the act itself, feeling one's self for pleasure or relief, whatever you may want to say about it, I was always afraid to talk about the subject but I found woman do it all the time and talk about it like it's nothing, most really do have vibrators in there draws, I was surprised at the difference with woman on the level of openness, everything intimate is talked about, so now I can! And where if you grow up a male, it's a sign you are weak you will not be a man, but I feel ok as a woman I could do that for a man, and help take care of him and his needs, also It's what a boy does, not masturbating as the word but the way a boy has to, It is very different from the way woman do, If I picture myself as a woman and masturbating a man, I don't feel awkward, and would not be inhibited to help him relieve himself, And if I would To see two men together and one masturbate the other is a real turn off, Just like watching two men kiss I don't like it, I am very uncomfortable, I see two woman, I admit I like that, It may be that all my life I learned from my mother woman hate sex! And to see them explore is wonderful, and all my life I have only been with woman, I did not step over that boundary, as long as I had a penis, I said no! Seeing two woman together for myself has helped me take away the feeling woman don't like or want men for sex, and that they do not like to have sex at all that only men do, I was taught this all my life by my mother, seeing myself as a woman in my mind and masturbating with my own hands or sex tools does not make me feel awkward, know if I am a woman in the first place, and I want to feel like one, and also as all these years I have longed for a vagina and feel of a vaginal penetration, I would welcome it, I would feel like a woman even through masturbation, because I am one, and would not feel awkward I am not throwing a curve at myself, as being a woman in a man's body and having a penis, that's the curve, like I am in a man's body with a dress on trying to fool myself, no matter how deep I can get into any fantasy, with a penis attached to my body, there is always a connection to my brain that knows what my body is doing no matter how deep I can get into any fantasy, the same act, a simple up and down stroke with your hand on a penis my body and brain together know what it is doing to myself, I am assuming there are some that may be able to control that process much better, But me I never could, and I always felt to myself, That it was important that I don't do things sexually that will not come back later to depress me or make me feel guilty it's not worth it, this alone is enough to endure, one problem at a time, take care of your own heart first, so no your wrong about that, a real woman like myself in a man's body will not like to dress in woman's clothing just to masturbate, but deny that part of life as much as possible, and not because it is thought of as a bad thing to do or a shameful act, it's what a boy does, and you happen to be a boy and have a penis and really feel like you are a boy then you are going to really enjoy that, I have been around many boys growing up at the age of finding things out and things I saw and heard still shock me, so no! not all of us dress as woman and masturbate and fantasize at that moment we are a woman having intercourse, it's a myth, it's the last thing I want to do, in fact why wear the clothes if you are into a fantasy just use that! You can be in a clown suit and if you have a good imagination it will work just as well. Clothes have little to do with being a woman but when you are in the clothing that suits your gender it's an outer expression of your feelings you want to share not an inward feeling, I want to dress, look at myself for but a moment to see what I appear to be to others, that will look back at me, and that is a woman, I know I see now what others do and that's where I start to become myself, that's when I feel that I feel right coming out of me, I am ready to go out there and embrace the world feel my emotions in my search of my soul, not my penis, and it has always been like this, I have thought this way before and after puberty, it made no difference, puberty only made things worse I knew then, I was going to have a long hard lonely life, sex is the one area everyone is curious about, but sex is a programming in your brain, It starts early, before we even understand why, I believe guilt and religious beliefs play a part in how "I" will act out in life with the choices I make, and with who my family was, and who brought me up. I have read other books on this gender subject, where some feel nurturing plays a role in this development completely, but what I find with others like myself it is about eighty percent of what they have felt and gone through are a perfect match, never one hundred percent and that's where all that nurturing part comes in, as myself I was religious at a very young age "six" not any special name to it, like Jewish or catholic, I knew nothing of it, though we were raised catholic, I never associated myself to any group I just put my soul and life in gods hand, but I also had an actual spiritual experience, and having such an experience at such a young age and brought up in a strong Christian and god believing catholic family, and knew I had a soul of my own to protect at so young an age, I knew and believed there was a god! And there was a judgment, and we were made to create children as men and woman, there was a reason for the two differences, it was said god hated all homosexuals? I looked this up, I read the complete bible, god hated men that loved other men, as other men will love themselves become vain and love only men and not god, How true, men would love themselves more than god if they lost control, many have, God understands his creation well and those of us he put here with our handicaps whatever they may be, they are not mistakes, every one of them is a lesson for each soul, god has given the opportunity to come into his heaven by given out acts of kindness to those who need help, with as for myself the idea of man and a woman is so amazing, What god has created is a perfect plan, and a wonderful creation. I would not change a thing, god had it right, I see so much of the nature in what god has done, it's all so wonderful, just to pick a tiny flower from the ground on a warm spring day and explore each soft petal they look alike but not one is exactly the same just like people, And there are tiny worlds inside every drop of water, where does all this come from, I know there are rules we must follow in nature and with our choices in mating and love, So we do not harm ourselves, physically or emotionally, I was always consumed in my thoughts, of love and sex and mating, I found being confused about my gender made me go deeper into my soul and my sexuality more than probably most of us do and I believe others like myself must do the same, that is why there are so many suicides and no one knows why they did it, We lose our battles daily, I know now why I feel like a piece of me goes with someone when they commit this act, I wonder if it was that they thought like myself and kept it in and found no help, or had a problem that would get a door slammed in there face, either way it was not a subject they could discuss, or it was something that if they came out and told someone a lot of people would feel hurt, and if you are like me you would rather hurt yourself first, I decided to mate with the opposite of what I was physically, it was a boundary I made for myself and was unwilling to ever step over, and was so happy to this day I did, and where I have become super hypersensitive through this struggle, making a wrong choice in such a most intimate emotion of them all would be a disaster, Even to mate or even embrace and touch anyone again is a challenge and an absolute fear I now have, It will be a relationship that may end bad no matter how I am dressed, if I want an honest one, I went through many, many hard times of growing with the pain of sexual development, The sexual thoughts, and fantasies, and the pornography, was difficult to look at. Talk about and explore, I would look at a poster of a naked lady and all of a sudden. I was her looking out at me. I wanted to look just like her. It was embarrassing at first, I did not know what was going on, I would see pictures of sex acts, men with woman I would become the woman in the pictures. Everything films, pictures, magazines, woman walking down the street. I was one of them, I felt it! How was I going to ever have a normal relationship, what woman would ever really want me if they knew I harbored such a secret, the only real solution for me someday was to become a woman. I knew it! I knew I was born a woman inside a man's body, by now, it's more obvious than ever There is no other reason for any of this, it's very terrifying to realize this, there is no way out and you know nobody will want you and you learn that very young, and finally when you decide that, you know you don't need anyone else's opinion about what you are, all the things that you go back through from your toddler years up to your teens when you are hitting you pubescent period in life, and the stresses and strains of the emotional and physical changes, you go through are so overwhelming the only other way out may be suicide, and a lifetime of suicidal thoughts and fantasies can take over and give your ideas and solutions to your problem that you are going to harm yourself with, Children need help very early maybe not at eight or nine but, If they get up to thirteen fourteen and you hopefully have kept an eye on them, please help them, open your heart not your door, they may just disappear one day or night on you suddenly, not really wanting to die, it's not an act, it's been a cry for help, with no listeners, and the acts for attention finally end up killing your baby who really did not want to die but really wanted to live, no one who has such a loving spirit wants to destroy it. he or she only wants to share it, But is sometimes held back so hard and so long by our societies and medical rules of the world we live in, and our own families, and friends and the ones we want to love and love us back no matter what, I made two attempts and failed, when I was 17 and most of it came from the fear and all the misunderstanding I faced every day, when I woke up and decided, I want to be me, but I had to push the weight of the world off me first, so many of you have lost loved ones without an explanation of why they did it, don't be one of them, just be kind to everyone, that's all it really takes, and find love somewhere, and embrace it as long as you can, at least once, it will always be a reference point for your soul to find its direction, if you can do that than some and others going through the hell I went through, and still going through will be a little easier, remember it's someone that told you, they loved you, and you told them you loved them too, and they really meant it, they will never forget, ever! I am going to do an experiment with a chair this takes away the covers and blankets we hide under, and expose myself out in the light out in the open. To explore the intimate details of my sexuality separating fantasy from reality and opening myself up to what I would have to experience in the real world, and what I am willing to do and what boundaries I will and will not cross also remember I have lived as a man, I was born one, physically, And I have only in my life been with woman, so I have gone by my own instincts and experience and I want to show where it is in the sexual programming in my own brain that lets me do the acts and love making that I will let myself do, I seat the woman on this chair she is naked she can look at herself and me, I am now the male I see her, she is a beautiful woman, she sit's open to accept me. My penis swelling about to explode from anticipation and the feeling to dominate is very strong, when you are standing there as a man with a firm hard erection, the chemical reaction in your brain sends signals, to your brain, the feeling of wanting to dominate are more intense. as the warm soothing penetration deep into her! Is a few seconds of waiting that seems like long minutes, and the look of surrender on her face as I push into her and hold onto her ever so tight, and we start our rhythmic motion till we both orgasm I feel my own penis throbbing inside her, and her vagina grabbing my penis tightly I know I have pleased her, it's mutual, so much love, we are such loving creatures there are many things we can do sexually from a chair as in acts we do and can perform on each other. I can stand there and hold her soft cheeks in my hand and gently feel her face as I take her long hair into a ponytail and hold it not so firmly as I hold myself to her lips in hopes she will open and receive me, and do so willingly as if she wants to, There is also the feeling of power and domination as I am above this woman, I can use my strength to do what I want without being as gentle, I could use the strength nature gave me as an advantage to see that I succeeded in mating, I am letting her feel me any way she wants everything looks and feels natural as I myself look down at her, on the chair, I see her breasts and the curves of her body, I know I stand before a woman there is no doubt in my mind at all that who I am with is my sexual partner, and I enjoy the soft feel of her breasts and the look of pleasure on her face as my hands explore her soft warm body, It is what nature intended it is a beautiful moment of love and not just a moment of sex, and to see her take a hold of my penis and gently massage it, It belongs to her, and she holds with comfort and ease and a look on her face that makes me feel she needs me, and she needs me to need her, and wants to make that part of me enjoy it, and I am not afraid to let her hold me, but I must be honest to people who read this book who want to answer questions about my or their own sexuality, And what steps to take and are they willing to take them or not, and will I take them? People are curios, how would I handle being a woman and why not just go ahead and do things now? To be honest, I must place myself in the chair and become the woman and have a man stand in front of me do all

Cynthia Marie

the same things I have just described that I have done to her as a man, I will sit in this seat and I too am naked and I am a woman I have beautiful breasts and I look down, I see my curves and my womanly shapes, and I see this man standing in front of me, I am open to accept him, I can feel him reach for me and bring his penis to the entrance of my vagina and I look down and I see it about to plunge into it as he grabs me tightly, and pulls me in to embrace me ` in real life would I do this? yes I would, I don't feel any resistance nor do I feel it's wrong, and I have to go a little further and be brave and I know that we do other things in our love making, if he approached me and he feels my soft face with his hands. And he himself firmly pulls my hair into a ponytail like I just did to that woman myself, and he put himself to my lips with that look of domination on his face and hopes of me receiving him, would I open and receive him, the answer would be the same and the feeling of power I had as the man would be removed, it would be a feeling of surrendering not my body but my emotions as I embrace all of them in the moment, And I would only want to be a good woman for him, and he brings his penis to my hand to touch him would I feel that child hood inhibition, no! I would not I would want to help him and take care of his needs I would feel no inhibitions at all, and as he massaged my breasts and my warm soft body, I know he is doing this to comfort me and let me know he wants to be gentle at this moment for me, as a special time for the two of us, but if I where to look down as I sat on this chair and I was the one sitting and it was a man that approached me and I look down at myself and there is a penis attached to myself, I would not be on the chair long I would get off there, even if I was halfway to becoming a woman and had breasts that would not help me. I am out in the open to myself I see who I am and I can make that distinction about who and what I am, and it's important to be correct, with a penis still attached to me not even having to see it but feel it there I feel a need to dominate still, if there is an arousal, I do not want to be in encounters like that where I may want to dominate, I cannot benefit from them, it is a chemical reaction in my brain from arousal, I need to see myself as well as feel myself as a woman to fully appreciate the experience of the moment, emotionally the journey into becoming a woman is a journey into your emotions the sexual part is incomplete, if you yourself are incomplete also, if you are going to become a woman you are going to find it is a journey deep into your emotions and soul you never thought

82

possible, Every one of them is a flower, You will pick and look carefully at each petal and explore every detail of it, and you will find some not so pretty, and a few a little rough and thorny, it is not a bouquet of sexual adventures, if you go in that direction you will exhaust yourself. And maybe get stuck with thorns, and may miss the opportunity you had to look deep into your own heart because it was clouded in miss beliefs, dreams, and sexual fantasies that only lasted but a few moments and were not what you expected, you cannot fill in the blanks yourself, as you cannot tell someone what a rose smells like if they never had one, they have to hold one themselves and smell it, it will be the same with sex, if you use fantasy in place of reality you will lose what you are really looking for, yourself, You have to be honest with yourself at the beginning of your journey, no one can tell you what interests you, you know your own needs, we need to love as a species and it comes out of the need to make a new life, And you must put those two together, it will keep you in a positive direction and not cause you to drift side to side, it will only confuse you and later in life. It may come back to haunt you when you are all alone, and you are struggling with depression, just in case you are alone, you may be lucky, and find someone who loves "you" I hope that you can put yourself in a chair like I have done to myself and be naked and look at yourself close and also think as you sit, that others are looking also. To see how you will act as they will judge you on that, You must always consider and keep in the back of your mind that if you like me have been born with this gender that does not match your body, and you know your place is safest in a woman's body and it's where you will do best and survive, it is the right place, go there first and do the rest later, you will know what to do when the time comes, and you will be happy you waited, be most intimate to your heart first there is plenty of time for the other later, I liked using the chair in many examples for my own self as I developed and grew, it always exposed myself out in the open I had to be honest to myself and anyone looking in, Even when I think back as a young boy and I had trouble with puberty the chair was useful not then but now thinking back, I did not have this idea then, but I wish I had, it opens up all relationships I would or anyone else may encounter, if I was a man and was in that chair and another male came in the room it would mean get out, two cannot dominate at the same time, I have no idea why two men would have sex together, I am not gay so I cannot take you there, to me it does not make any sense, working and playing alongside with men like I have done, I have only seen a hard side of them, never a gentler side, only in myself I have seen that, and a small hand full in my lifetime, and what I have read and heard it's not so gentle an act between the two men, and if one will want to dominate the other it can be a little violent, when the other decides he wants his turn to dominate, I knew a few couples and they were all much the same, but I cannot tell you they are all like that I am not gay, and I cannot explain to you what two men are seeking, also that I am as confused about that as I am myself, so I understand and respect them for their feelings and the pain they must endure like myself to be accepted, but also I am not a man emotionally only physically and it would not work to have a relationship with a male he would want me to keep my penis and I myself do not and the relationship would end, we are two different sides of the coin, and over the years on hormones that has changed a lot. I am more physically female now, what little bit of a man I have left is like taking the stem off an apple, I wondered if I was with someone like myself who was as gentle as me. another person born in a males body but a woman, I believe, if he was truly like myself we would struggle over who would be the wife in the relationship, neither would want to really be the husband, we would make a sweet couple if we got along, and certainly I know that in any man I would consider to seek I would look for that quality, I am a woman I just had some tiny mishap at birth, Something went wrong with the outside, inside I am perfectly normal as a woman, I found in real life, love making to some woman was difficult, They would say they feel like there in bed with another woman. I was to gentle, they missed the rougher male side that I did not have or found difficult to bring out, I assumed woman wanted a gentle touch, but not all do, and too find a woman who would like to be with someone like me is difficult, I myself decided I wanted to be with a woman always, I have always been with them and I need their love and nurturing still and I am scared and very lonely out here, Even without my surgery I don't feel I have any desire to dominate her if I become erect anymore, and that is something that would have to wait till the tears stop first, no woman is going to have the patience for me, I am someone lost in the middle and I am someone no one really wants, and feel lucky to be with anyone at all, if I am so lucky to have a moment to embrace a woman again it will be me that's surrenders, I am only so thankful that such a loving being will take me in and hold me close as I cry away fears of being rejected, that I may scare her away with to gentle a touch, I would not even like to push my own penis in, I would want her to hold it and guide me into her and help pull the two of us together, that way I feel it is her taking me and not me taking her it would be more mutual and both wanting, and if I can still please her I would be a truly happy woman, but I still always remember this a journey that most likely if taken it is one taken alone, No one is coming with you everyone in your life stands back and watches, you are going to walk that line in between everyone for a long time and you are going to scare most of them away, as gentle as you are and as kind as you will be becoming they will see only a monster growing, and most will not change, people who you thought would be the most trusting will not be, and the ones you thought would turn on you right away may not, and be the first to give you a warm hug, It is full of surprises, Don't play with any of it, take all of it seriously because they do, and they are the ones who cannot decide what you are, not you, you know what you are, a woman! But to them, you are in the middle, you to them are an IT, and to those people you will always be an IT. If they know who you are they will never let you forget your place, and when you make mistakes they wait for you to fail.

It will only be worse if it is what you know you really needed to do, and gave up for them, it is a hard world as it is and enough hate and prejudice all around but you are right there in the front lines if they know you are transgendered be honest to yourself all the time you are the only one who will be, so don't take chances, Especially with love and romance, and intimate sex and relationships, it may not be you, you are hurting, and your journey to becoming a woman will be cluttered with the pain of others you have brought along with you, or left behind, and you will have enough to bare on your own, do not try to bring anyone with you unless you are very lucky, And have an open, up front relationship that can work. Right at the beginning, and not stop not even hesitate for anyone, always move forward, backsliding is very difficult, and very exhausting, I hope you will do well, we all go through rocky relationships but this one is the rockiest road a person can travel and a fight so hard just to find peace inside your own self, I would accept the punishment whatever it may be from god, But I also would accept fully my role as a woman. No matter what it be and there is so much more to it than "sexual acts", I have found that being a woman "sex! Is a small part of what you will face with your emotions? As they all grow on you so much heavier than men, sorrow, heart breaks, and the loss of loved ones, will tear holes through your heart and leave scars forever, Things men just bounce off like a leaf blowing in the wind, Men have their way to grieve and let it go, but woman keep their loved ones and losses in a safe little place inside of their hearts, that's what is so special about them we take for granted, I only hope my experience is helpful to anyone one who is thinking about making this change in their lives.

The parents and doctors who may read this I hope you can help someone in your life with their choice, I am fifty seven now, I am old! I know that when I do complete this transition the chance of a real relationship is not very good, practically zero and it has been so long now. I was seven years old when I opened that box in the attic and put on my first dress a little makeup and blush, it was fifty years ago, and twenty five years after opening that box that I sat in a doctor's office to start a conversation, to even start talking about where I was and what I should do, It's a long time and I am still struggling needlessly to complete my journey, my only obstacle now is the money for the operation itself or I would already be done, I would be a complete woman and be able to run away from the word "IT", and my true feelings are. that if and when I do and was ever so lucky I had someone just that special in my life, That one time I could embrace and experience the full complete pleasures of everything a woman I can, I hope I have a chair, because I think I would like to sit for that one, But the real truth is I don't expect it, I expect to be alone I waited too long and for me back then when I was a child, there was no help at all, I would most likely have to pay an expert to give me that one night I would need to make that experience as complete as I can, I still do not think it would be the same, I have found this journey to become a woman more deeper than I ever imagined and it is, what I tell you, it is, it is a journey into your emotions, not your sex, or sexual activity, but deep into your soul, sex will become a minor part of it when you get this far in, But you will not know that till you get here, I never thought of the consequences that it would have on my own heart, ` It aches and it has pains I never thought it could have, I always knew I was born a woman in a man's body but without the hormones and new experiences I have had what I thought before is very minor to what really happens, when as a teen my thoughts

I was a woman in a man's body although as right as I was, getting to this point in my life now is an experience I never imagined, I was just an infant at that time compared to what I am now, and if you love and can embrace those feelings and emotions then you are on your way, you will be able to do anything from there, just get there first before you do the rest, my hardest part was I brought someone with me and found out she were not in it with her heart or it was not what she thought it would be, and she realizes how much now she has married a woman and not a man, although I did my best to warn her and tell her. myself that young, I did not either I always hoped that love would find a way in and make the scales balance, but love has to be honored on both sides and be very true and very mutual, or it will not work, in my lifetime there was no help, no one to go to, no supporting parents or friends, teachers, doctors, some girl next door, there was no one, I had only myself to gage and my own self to rely on and my own soul to protect, my own experiences to watch and care for. As a child any mention of it meant I may be punished. Ridiculed, even institutionalized just for saying I feel a little different to the wrong person, I am happy that the newer and younger generation can get information, and get help earlier in life, I only hope the medical field and health insurance company's open their minds and their hearts to people like myself who struggle there entire life needlessly for a simple answer, too! Help me! I would have made many different choices and not brought people I tried to love that I have hurt along the way And you must think of them first as you go along, If not then you are not becoming the woman you seek to be, you will become a woman if you really want to, go to Thailand if you got ten thousand dollars they will turn you into one, but an ordinary one at best with no real experience with your emotions, and then learn from your mistakes finding out you made a bad choice, and want your penis back, You may feel you mutilated yourself, why bother, when you can embrace all there is to take in as you prepare, so much that you will feel like one without the surgery, That's when you are ready for that last step, that's what I wanted, and that's where I am today, my case I have children and I must stop and slow down and back step many times causing my own distress and emotional conflicts they do not understand, I now have to start a new search for a gender therapist, and the next doctor I meet handled gender issues in a different approach, more of what I hoped for and I needed, I had come to a point I was physically breaking down, my heart was racing to the point of nearly passing out, and I was having seizures and, panic attacks, and that damn depression just hung like a noose around my neck daily, as if I wore a shadow necktie, All I wanted to do was die, or find a way to do it, without pain, all my thoughts where depressing thoughts of people I love dying all around me, friends and myself, I was consumed in daydreams and thoughts of everyone including myself dying or being killed I had no peace in my mind at all, The first therapist was not good, His idea to make me happy as a man first then work on the woman part later did not sit well, I already did that, I could stop right now and go back, It would be easier to be a man, I have already done that, and I was doing it well that was not my problem I found the therapist and had found my first real step into becoming a woman, life was not to be the same again ever, But as I am waiting for my appointment to approach I get a phone call, it is her, a friend from the past I have always held onto and never let go of, it's hard to let go of something as a pleasant and wonderful a memory, when you find you are alone and scared and the world has emptied you out of its heart and thrown you into solitude because you just don't fit, she lived a few towns over and I asked if I may visit, we met for about an hour, she had a young daughter and a baby in a crib and was alone, in the middle of a separation or some dispute, we just caught up a little with our lives, and had a nice catch up discussion, and I told her I would get back soon to see her again I had left and returned a few weeks later to tell her what I was planning and was going to see a doctor to start my program, and I wanted to tell her everything I was doing, a part of me was hoping she could say something, anything at all to give me an idea of what I should do, and if I should go into this reassignment program I would have loved to have her blessing, but when I went to see her she was gone, she had suddenly moved, the emptiness of the apartment and the darkness inside making all the windows look so black, left me feeling the same in my heart, all alone and empty. A feeling I know all too well, and hoping where ever she went, she was going to be ok, I go into a life changing moment forever, I go see my new therapist we met first for six months, I took written tests was asked a series of questions. Was observed, I just did what I was asked told everything truthfully, and let myself feel natural, I hid no feelings, and was found to be high up on the scales of the BEM test, a test that measures you gender with a series of questions you must answer honestly as some are trick questions, and scored high as having a female mind, and thought very much like one, I already knew that, but it was good to see results on paper, he told me he was excited to have me as a client and that if I go all the way with him I would be his first documented case start to finish, He had starts who moved away and finished later and he had others who had already started somewhere else and then finished, One year or so after I start with the therapy he persuades me to join a support group and one night a week I met with many others like myself, there again was a whole world out there, I was not so alone, and I was away from the home and had my day to some peace of mind. There are so many men that love to wear a dress, my god is there, but I had found in the support groups "my" numbers where low, Most where cross dressers only, part time girls, they don't want to be a girl or woman full time, they like going home or back to the office in their male role and be the boss, the man again, and I find sometimes I conflict with some of them, they get persistent that I should be like them, stay a man, stay in charge, just get out once and awhile and have some fun and relax, get the stress out, I wonder how many of them where the boys in line with me in first grade saying something similar about it being better to be the boy and made fun of girls and being one, and made fun of boys who wanted to be one, and learned themselves later getting into a nice dress once and a while was a blast, I met one that cross dressed once a year only, she did not know why, I saw her sitting alone on a chair she was a knockout, I could not believe she was that good at makeup doing it that little and she dressed real nice, you would never know she was a he ever, she told me it's just once a year, I have to get it out of my system, I have no idea why, I don't see a therapist, my girlfriend has no idea, I just need one day a year and it's over, I learned fast I was not a cross dresser, and it got to a point I got so annoyed by some who would not stop telling me to go part time, I dropped my support group, in that time I was there I only met a few like myself, how amazing it is to talk to someone just like you, and I will not meet many but when I do I enjoy every second we talk, we almost read each other's minds, I also wanted to start hormones many were talking me out of it, don't do it, you will regret it, everyone will know, your secret will be out, but I know what I want. I want female hormones running through my blood whether they worked or not, I am a female, my life will be out, it's not a secret, it has been a reality that others keep me from becoming, it would be there secret if

Cynthia Marie

they had it there way, but if you want to really live, then don't keep
secrets, secrets like anything else get around and when they do by the
time it gets back to you it's a whole new story, but also finding others
in my support group was a good thing for me it showed how the world
and people are so diversified and the many degrees in a person's gender
and their own orientation to it, both man and woman, we had a female
to male come in and I was not told, I was just told he was a visitor and
had to be screened, I thought he was waiting for someone to come in
and screen him for the correct security questions, as a male to female,
and they are simple but I can't say what they are, it's like knowing the
password to get in, I had no idea it was a female to male and he was
already in his male persona so I thought I had to wait for the right
person, for a male to female, it was the clubs first venture into opening
up to both, he looks and reminds me he has been there awhile and he
thought he would get accepted right in and he came with friends, even
still he had to get the screening questions, and I said you certainly are
accepted here, and I go get someone and find out what is really going
on, I was upset and embarrassed for myself the transgendered person
and the friends who brought him, I blasted them, I told them he has sat
there all this time because no one came and told me, and is out there
feeling rejected, I just went in and told him my confusion and that I and
the club apologize for this, I should have been told by who walked you
in the door right then, they know the rules, I said just go inside and
meet everyone you don't need to talk to anyone just go in, and I am
sorry for the delay, but you fooled me, I really thought you were a man
coming to get screened, no one told me, after that they made sure bad
communication like that would not be tolerated, and it's my first time of
the receiving end of being fooled, my therapist found me a doctor for
the hormone therapy and being married my wife had to sign a waiver to
allow me to take them, understandable, there were going to be some
changes, and they would come very quick and very natural to me, It
was like my body was missing them all this time, just like vitamins. my
mind fell at peace, for the first time in years, I rode a bicycle on an old
path at a park and it was the first time I felt my breast bouncing up and
down, they were still small, but what a feeling that was, I hit every
bump I saw, I had waited so long to feel that, and it's something a few
years ago, that I never thought I would have felt, I only imagined it as I
watched other girls ride or run through parks, and now it was me, I was

becoming a girl, a woman soon, and I was in heaven at that moment, but all the horrors where to soon come, the hate and the discrimination, and abuse. I was to take for many, many long, long years from friends and family, it is so sad strangers treat you better than your own, and if you even get past the first two or three years you will make it but it does not even end there, it is a long road of hate and rejection that you will endure for a lifetime, so if you are thinking of this change in your life be prepared for that, And be very sure, and don't wait till your old, get a good young start, 14-15, even thirteen if you really got a lot of people to love and help you in your family, and you won't get thrown out into the cold, how I began my steps and with the way my therapist and how doctors advised, And started my program was wrong, learn from the mistakes made here so you don't suffer the many tears and years of hurt to yourself and others like I did, following old rules and being too hard on yourself. The first step is in the beginning is if you can accept that every day you will cry out with such grief like never before, as if your body gets to a point it's just peeing out water from your eyes, and it can last days even weeks, at anytime, anywhere, anything that brings a hurt feeling picks you up and carries you off like a big large wave, you cannot escape it, you would never in your life believe that a human can cry so much, less than starving children and those whose backs are broken by their masters, then you can start, but that is the first and easy part, your first baby step into becoming a woman, accept that crying will become so much a part of your life that after you have embraced your womanhood, you realize that you cannot live without it. And that your emotions and feelings are on their way to growing and making you a more spiritual being than you ever imagined your journey would take you into, never mind so much the physical change as so much as the emotional ones that will take you over, and if you can embrace it, love it, and begin to enjoy every tear that falls, Then you are on your way to becoming a woman. When I got my prescription finally for my hormones I had to pay for them myself, as the health insurance back then was not paying anything at all, for any part of this, The name of a male on a bottle of female hormones raised a lot of eyebrows at the pharmacist I had used for the last ten years, but I was did not care I knew them all so long and they were nice people. I was going to see if they stayed like that, and they have! I still go there, taking my first hormone gave me a feeling of taking a ticket on a train ride I would be going on, and I would be up front all alone driving and the hormone was the ticket to get on the train, I remember my very first mammogram I would get. It would be with my male name, the receptionist asked why do you need a mammyogram I said I guess it's a routine mammyogram I do not know what the doctor ordered, she said ok. Then a nurse comes out five minutes later and wiggles her finger, come here, she says, she gets me in a room and shuts the door and say's ok what's up here, tell me! it's ok I have heard it all, I need to know why you are here, don't be scared to talk, I just came right out and told her, she did not blink an eye, she said I thought so, I have a friend who is doing this, good for you, That was so good my first female exam and my first mammogram even though it was not pleasant I still loved it, I was hoping everything would go that well but I am afraid not, and the hormones themselves, just taking that first one even though it was to do anything, made me feel like I was going to be ok, I was going to finally be a girl. and girl hormones where now running through my blood, I was about 35 years old and I was finally coming to life, and I really understood that I had to start slowly and I would be a girl first, then a woman, I had to grow that way, I knew I would not just become a woman in just a year or two like magic, I knew it would take time to experience my knew emotions and feelings and learn to adapt to those of my loved ones around me, no one had to tell me either this was not my therapists idea, it was my own, as I grew and developed and when I looked at it that way, it made it a little easier, I made mistakes a lot, I knew I was just learning, I was a long way to becoming a woman, My age meant nothing I had to approach it as if I were a young girl starting out and beginning puberty and growing into a woman, and it was a very helpful approach, I found it easier not to be so hard on myself knowing that I was still only a young girl who needed a lot of experience, before I felt I would even myself be able to finally say to myself I have made it, and through my life I have been so hard on myself but for other people, I need to be kind to me, myself now I am tired of the abuse I even got from my own self trying to please everyone else, the people around you do not see a young girl starting out. they see you as an adult and they automatically assume you are a grown adult woman, and you are no way even close, you have a long way to go, within a few months I felt pain in my breast and they grew little small round circles, and I felt weight and pressure around them, there was not much really showing but I felt them developing, I waited a lifetime to feel that and now here it was, And it was as wonderful as I had hoped, I was still working as a tool and die maker, and really did want to wait several years before I had alerted anyone or wanted to make a decision to come out, I had time, I always wore a shop coat so no one would ever see any changes and I would just go about life like nothing was changing, but a bad back caught up to me, tool and Die work is hard on your back, I went to my boss and told him I got hurt lifting a shoe onto a milling machine, It's heavy precise vise to hold parts in so you can cut them. Or hold them while you put in a precision hole pattern in a steel block, I got x-rayed and was told my back was as bad as an eighty year old man's back, several fractures and slipped and bulging discs from my tail bone up to my neck and arthritis has fused many vertebrae together, some looked congenital and also it appeared at one time I had fractured my back where it meets the hip, and very hard to detect, it must have been twenty years old or more but they said physical therapy would be a big help, so I said I would do it, I had massages stretching exercises small weights, and electrical muscle stimulating heat pads, I loved that! I want those at home, and soon they suggested to get into a pool to help get my strength back sooner, I was having trouble recovering, and did not know why, and later would find it was a genetic muscle disease in the family and not the injury itself causing it, but it was brought out by the injury. and complicated healing and where they were not doctors, and could not find anything wrong with me also, At the occupational clinic, they treated me like I was faking my injury to stay out of work longer, But when I had an EMG done by a neurologist they sent me to and a genetic muscle disease showed up, They looked embarrassed they treated me that way, I was right! Something was really wrong with me, so I said ok to a few trials in the pool. And I had felt safe, my breast really weren't growing yet, I did not think any of the guys would notice but a few woman did, they know what a breast looks like going through its pubic stage, and I did not, yes I have daughters and sisters but I never really looked, there my daughters and my sisters. It never occurred to me ever to look at them. And watch their development, why would I? There my daughters, it's not something I would just look at and study on my own children or any other child, that feels so wrong, I am very cautious with those things my oldest daughter had trouble with her son potty training and asked I helped and I told her I couldn't, He was not my son, just being a grandchild makes that much difference to me I cannot and will not ever cross that line, It is not my child or responsibility, I told her it was up to her to solve that herself, "she sat on a lot of wet toilet seats", I felt bad he got yelled at by all the woman in the house, when he visited, but there was nothing I could do, I believe only a parent should see their child in those matters, unless they are no longer alive, then I may reconsider, only in a medical book I had seen what development looked like but it was not the same in real life, And when I was being examined two woman came in together giggling and saying how do you like our new "man" patient this "man" has a hurt back I and they giggled and one left the room, and at first I wondered what the joke was, she came back in looked at my chest and backed out again, laughing, oh god they noticed, I looked down and I even had noticed a slight curve upward had started, My god I was so embarrassed, but I still thought it was a mistake, some men have large ones similar to this, only they are heavy I was not I was still pretty firm and my muscles were firm my six pack was still there, but I had no hair it was coming off me, my chest lost hair fast, I came back one more time, hoping it may be some office joke, It's not me they are laughing at, I am in the pool and I notice a lot of people men and woman are now watching me exercise. And I look down at my chest and they seem to protrude outward from the cold water. That's what it was, it was the cold water, they popped right out, unlike the male penis that does the opposite, when in cold water hides like a frightened turtle, my breasts came right out, like a fourteen or fifteen year old girl and did not look like man boobs at all they had that nice curvy girly shape. I looked a topless woman in the pool. I was so embarrassed. I got right out, dressed and never went back, we had an occupational nurse at work then but I went to my gender therapist first to explain to him what happened and what I should do. I did not want to go back to physical therapy. I wanted to get back on full duty and off light duty but I need to explain why I don't want to go back and that I feel ok to work. She appears to be a very nice woman, I tell my therapist I may need to talk to her about it, and he says well it may be a good time to tell someone in your company where you are at this point. After all if you will be staying there during the complete transition, And at the time it was a plan to stay, and you feel you have a safe person to confide in, then give it a try and see what happens, I do, and she is at first very surprised but seems to take it well and seems very happy for me, A few days later she returns she said she spoke to the occupational doctor at the clinic and was told my back was so bad that I would have to remain on light duty permanently, But no pay cut, and that I would still get increases in pay. So what could I do, I need to stay working, and I am giving a desk job, But telling someone at that point (was bad) and way to early, my therapist should have said wait, tell the clinic you are better and take it from there, I needed directions and ideas, too much was going on in my life and making decisions was very hard I wish I had waited, I learned fast people cannot be trusted and my therapist should have protected me a little bit more being so soon into my program with him, she had gone to the president of the company and he said take me out of the tool and die shop, the men won't like it, but I never knew who she told, she acted like a good friend and a person I could trust, but she was not, she took my career away out of prejudice, and I would learn just how far that went through this company although they say they want to help, they really don't, and myself I was an anxious girl waiting to explore, I was just starting on hormones, and unprepared for the emotional shifts that were coming, my therapist really should have said that to me, I also have a family life at home the wife the kids, the changes in all our lives, that will be coming, my oldest was 17 and getting out of control and hanging with a bad crowd, many nights we went out looking for her in dangerous parts of the city when her so called friends abandoned her, and left her alone in the dark cold streets of the inner city, although As tough as she acted, when it really came to gang banging her heart just wasn't in it for real, but she brought home one hell of a bad boyfriend, a black kid, It was cool to date a black guy then, rapping was the new thing if you were a white chick with a black boyfriend you were cool, and my daughter was so in to being cool and showing off, and he said he was a "rapper" and that girl she hung with was also into them, And got my daughter also, later she would regret it, she has a son from him and tells everyone he is every ethnic race there is except what he really is, African American, They look at her like she has two heads, He had his own little CD in his pocket bragging he was always hanging at the studio and going to get signed, my foolish naive daughter believing it all and drooling over this halfwit. I remember Paragon Park in hull Ma, for fifty cents you could go in booth play music on a karaoke type machine sing into it and put in on a 45 single and go tell your girl you were getting a singing contract. What an old routine and here is my daughter falling for it? I warned her and warned her but no, she would not listen. That's the one real special thing I had to give my daughters, was telling them what to watch out for and how to tell bad men from the good ones, And I could help them make decisions when they asked and needed advise I gave the honest answer to protect them from harm, but my oldest wanted to do whatever she wanted and paid no attention to any advice I would give her, and the relationship with this boy would bring three years of absolute hell never mind the sex change, this was something altogether different that would intertwine and blow things so far apart that in the end I would lose my relationship with my oldest daughter forever, The first night I meet him is on Halloween night, I get a call at work from my wife that my oldest daughter has a close friend that got arrested and needs to be bailed out can we help? I said what for? Why was he arrested? She said armed robbery? I said armed robbery? Yes, she replies, armed robbery, but he didn't do it, he is being framed by some old girlfriend. I said no! She said it's only 5000.00 we have it at the moment, I said 5000.00? what are you? Out of your mind? You don't even know what really happened, and you don't even know him, leave him there till you find out more of the facts, she says ok, I come home, there he is all set for trick or treat, she bailed him out anyway.

And I was horrified when I met him, and not because he was black, but so nervous, every time a car drove by He swayed and ducked and watched, And I said what are you doing that for? And he said, drive by man, I said drive by what? He said drive by! You know in da hood! People they just drive by and shoot you. Don't matter what! They just shoot, they think you someone else, or someone they want to get even with, they don't care, they pull out there gun and just start shooting, I just think to myself my god my daughter is with this! What the hell am I going to do? And her friends are horrible one a girl so bad that before she is twenty one every reproduction organ in her body will have been removed. From all the STD's she has had, I came home one day from work years ago she and my oldest daughter came into the house with this girl. My wife did not want her in the house, and kept telling them to get out, my own daughter came up behind her own mother and hit her to the side of her face so hard with a closed fist she needed 38 stitches inside her mouth, the hospital thought I did it, but was shocked to hear who really did, and why they did not call the police I will never know, only that her mother protected her and said she was going too, they never should have let her or anyone make that decision, abuse like that needs to be nipped in the butt, right away, and this was just the beginning of the hell I would face with my daughter as I move ahead into my transition, years later, this was going to be harder than I thought, not the sex change as much as the sex change with a daughter like this, I started having severe panic attacks so severe they thought I was having seizures, I felt like I was dying, and I started on depression medicine and other medicine to soften the panic attacks, And depression always just tagged along any ways, always there, sometimes just a better day than the other but it was always there, It started so long ago it just embedded itself in my soul. I had become so loss of all my feelings, that sadness and grief were ones that could keep coming in and fill the emptiness, wrapping itself around me like a warm blanket. Drifting away into suicidal thoughts. Planning them out became so routine that it became jthe only feeling I had left, except hope, hope has a feel, like anticipation without the nervousness, something may come along but it may not, but you knew the feel of it while you waited, it was that little stick in the pile that if you pull it out they all fall down, you don't know where it is or how to find it, you just wait till it comes along and finds you, and tears always if I had thought I had had enough from just being depressed I was in for a real surprise when I discovered, that the changes in my own emotions from the hormones created a pms like symptom but far worse, it lasts longer, months sometimes. If you go off your routine and slide off your scales then you develop pms till everything settles again, you are all over the place with your emotions, you always have the pms but it is well controlled if your meds are, Careful in between doctors if it should happen things can get very scary, but also there is a good side I don't want to scare you away from hormones if you need them, the happier side of the pms is there also, that glow that woman get when they are pregnant or in love. or have that little crush, those moments the flowers look so much prettier and smell so much more beautiful, happen also, hold onto those moments closely guard them, keep them in your memory and in your heart and grow from them, they get better and they are the ones that will rescue you and balance you out and keep you going to find that inner strength, these are the ones that will become so deep and alive as you go along that you will be so happy you did not give up, but at home my oldest daughter was just taking control of the house, with force and threats, she comes to me and tells me she will do anything she wants, and if I tell her no! she will call the dss and say I beat her, when I heard that, my heart sank, I saw nothing but trouble ahead and at the time she assaulted her mother I wish we had done something more drastic to wake her up and give her a dose of reality, Let her see what she really had, go in and have to share a television with a bunch of girls your age who don't like what you like And you have to be in bed at 9:00 pm. sharp every night, worry about finding your shoes or those nice jeans you had in the morning when you wake up, a little boot camp experience, We would regret it later we never did she was a kid who needed that, She was in so much trouble and so arrogant that she made her threat real, by coming to the home with a friend of hers and is asked to leave, they refuse, I go up to her room and go over to her while she lies in her bed and she kicks me right in the stomach, I grabbed her foot while it's sunk into my stomach, I pull her off the bed and say get out, her friend already long gone, get together work out a scheme smack her around a little, take her to the hospital and say I beat her up. And a nurse calls me screaming at me, and I say who is my daughter with right now, and she tells me, and says my daughter will be going home with them, she is not safe in your home, I say that boy right there that you are about to let my daughter leave with instead of sending her home, is a convicted child molester, and even though she checks my story and proves I am right and I say don't you get it? they are all up there lying, they hit her to make it look like I did, but she will not admit she is wrong and calls the police on me, that all ends well but that nurse should have lost her job, as far as I am concerned, And this is the daughter I have to deal with as I go into this transition, that she knows nothing of yet, she has never even seen me or knows I have cross dressed, the other two I have are going to be ok, but this one is just refusing to accept anything she doesn't want, or like, and will make another twenty years of my life hell Till we finally just have to say goodbye, I only wish her well, she was such a great baby, sweet smart kind, and a kid you knew would be anything she put her mind to, when we talk about nurturing in our lives and some say nurturing can make a person what they come out be, some say raise a young boy as a girl and he will grow into it. How wrong is that! But children are also nurtured outside in their neighbor hoods out with their friends and enemies finding their places. Once inseparable become their own little built family and they come home, someone you did not bring up, they have changed, they have brought along pieces of the identity of the ones outside the home they feel are there family, Manners outside the home into yours not always that it's bad, not all children are evil but if you lose your child to the ones that are of bad seed and it also goes for the parenting that these children that are out there to hurt us all, that uninvited trouble comes to your door and into your own home, These children in the project we moved to where everywhere not as bad but almost, and there were a lot of good ones, but it seemed my daughter was drawn to the loners, the kids who had little or nothing. Maybe she felt sorry, or maybe she just wanted to show off she had the best clothes, we were third highest in income in that project, So my children did well And at times we helped neighbors in need, when they had times they were just down on their luck, and all that part of it was nice, but the darker element of the children, who went about with souls that need love and attention are walking out there abandoned, just as shadows show themselves at night and daytime they are always there, and my daughter befriends many, it's amazing to me that she never figured out why her clothes where always missing, Never to be found, Was she that naive or was she in her way helping her needy friends at our expense, and then at the age of 17 she tells me she is pregnant, I tell her I would help her, and not to give up on this new life, my hope was this 22 year old boy would now become a man, yes 22 I find I was lied to, no surprise to me, I was told he was eighteen, I also had found out too. that some of my daughters expensive jewelry and nice leather coats I bought for her were on other girlfriends of his he hung at the studio with, And was finding out he had about 3-4 other children, his count to this date as I write this book last I heard was 14, one he may have had with a girl at the home of a friend who went out to shop and left him there to watch his little sister, I hear the baby looks just like him, but back then we tell her, all her good friends tell her, she will not listen to any one and loses many good friends, I even could have pressed charges she was a minor he was twenty two, But I know my daughter would only defend him, I was a color guard "dad" I like (soccer mom) I took all my kids every weekend Saturday and Sunday to their shows where they performed all over the state, and had won very high place trophies many times, we did this almost ten years. I videotaped for our team as they practiced during the week to help us win, if I couldn't drive I made sure they had all the money they needed for the bus they would rent, But when the guard my oldest daughter was in was going world, and she had leads in it, her worst of friends steered her away and from there into a life of destruction and misery that brought it all to an end, At home work still was at first ok the job load was very busy and I worked with two other woman one a much younger girl and an older woman, they were very nice and we all did our jobs, As a team it all seemed good. I developed a very close relationship and worked at letting them feel I was just a normal regular guy I just want to fit, and not get observed, And not make them feel because I am a man they have to change or say anything they do different, I was just me, quiet and polite, and I kept the craziness at home, police at my house constantly, when I arrive or being told by neighbors, my oldest daughter is being beaten again or loud outside and being abused by this boyfriend, And she is in that beginning cycle of it's her fault please come back, I am wrong I deserved it, to a point when I try to physically intervene I would be attacked from behind and by of all people my own daughter, and the police they walk in and actually see a big 225 lb. black man pinning down a young woman and it must be the cop who usually goes to get the donuts instead of making a domestic like this, all he will say is, get off her!, then leave, and make no arrests, all alone and now I am the one in trouble, I am the bad guy just for interfering, But as for me I have an ace in my pocket my confidence card, it's what got me here and will carry me along always it will give me a strong yet beautiful feminine walk also, so confident when I go into a room people notice, I am going to take control, why? Because I can, I have become a very powerful weapon, I have exercised and conditioned and molded my body into a weapon, from a style of martial arts known as Uiechi-Rye (the Chinese system) very rare style to be found, It was a matter of luck I had found this unique system from my good friend Bill, He helped someone fix a car and befriended him and told him of the school, it has the exercise of San Chin, they are what we in America call isometrics, but what we learn in this country is a cheap watered down copy, what I had the privilege to learn was a gift, a lot of the same Okinawan styles of Uiechi-Rye had San Chin, But it was not as complete, most of the 2 hour exercises alone was just the exercise of San chin which was about 1 and a half hours alone where in most other schools it is about ten or 15 minutes and watered down and changed, they will tell you it is not, but my teacher said not to listen, I was an exceptional student, but the school closed not enough students to stay open, It takes a long time to develop any strength and it looks and seems boring to learn to the casual observer who was interested in learning a martial art, from there I went on to study the other arts of Jujitsu, Kenpo, and Kung Fu. And along with the part of Uiechi-Rye after the exercises, the style of fighting was Chinese boxing not a lot of kicking, it was developed by the Chinese who worked in the rice patties. And they were always up to their waste in water, and to defend themselves made various hand arm elbow strikes, and blocks, and a technique of where one puts all its energy into an area of a person's body with a snap, and pull away leaving the energy in need of a place to go, and being so much force it will damage internal organs, sometimes the damage not felt or noticed for days. This technique is deadly and not used in sport karate, and it is not to be taken for granted as if you would to pull out a gun. it had better be for a reason to use it, and I learned it all well 15 years of 4-6 hours a day working out, I was like a piece of steel, I didn't look like it, either and I acted mild and meek, I was a sleeper, just like my friends old hot rods only it was myself, I was in so many fights growing up and when developing my skills along with others like myself going out back behind a building or off in the woods to practice, to develop our skills with no referee. Just a good fight, friendly but serious, we honed in our skills; as if we were a special breed, it was a sport I loved not so much for the fighting but the idea that it was a game of high speed chess and if you make a wrong move you get hit, and exercising all the time was very good to do, and here my daughter's boyfriend believes he can challenge me! all I say is if you are now prepared to die than just come here, I am not going to fight you, punch you around, kick you, nothing like that, if that's what you are expecting, I am just going to "kill you", and that is today, you are going to be dead today if you come near me, He said what? I said I will kill you! I don't stutter! And I am not playing! take a step over here and if you don't believe it come and try your luck, and first if you like, say any last prayer to any god you like to it will be your last, And I was serious this was going to happen, I had absolutely no fear what's so ever, the beatings and fights I got into all my life, are nothing to me now, the pain of a kick or a punch was as routine as eating lunch. And to the reader I am not trying to convey I am trying to be a man, no! It is, that I am really trying to protect my family, my daughter, and my two other children, and using the talents and skills I developed along the way to cope and try and adjust myself someplace in this world so I would be comfortable and not be scared, Self-defense training is great for that, I recommend you do study and learn yourself to take care of yourself in any way that you can, does not matter the style or where it comes from, learn to defend yourself, many woman are raped and beaten and abused needlessly, and right now it is a lesson learned, This monster backed down and ran away, and honestly it surprised me, I really thought he would try and I was not bluffing either, it was going to happen if he came near me, I had taken bigger and better than him, this tough guy from the hood, ran from a fight, the true coward he is, his nature showed, It should have woken up my daughter, but it did not, let me tell you as surprised as I was, I was in a happy realization that how helpful all this training was and later the confidence I would have and the brave face it helped me keep in the worst of times and still does, I am old now 57 writing this, my back has completely collapsed, it hurts like hell I have days I can barely move and that's not all I have for disabilities, I have seizures, coronary artery disease! Angina, Charcot Marie tooth disease, restless leg syndrome, sleep apnea have had three strokes, CIDP, migraines, loss of 60 percent or more of my hearing, my neck to my tail bone has issues some congenital, and bad ones! fractures and slipped bulging disc some completely gone, And the vertebrae are touching down and grinding away and are fusing together, suicidal fantasies, depression, panic attack syndrome, and of course (gender dysphoria) on top of all this and there are a few more but I can't think of them they may come up later, But I have always just found that little bit of strength to keep pushing. That desire to complete myself is very strong, stronger than any of the tests and trials I have put myself through, I had to let out this woman inside me, she was really there, and she is "me", and where do I go from here? many books I read the writer would explain themselves as two separate people, but it was not that way for me, I did not like that separation, it was a split in half feeling, and I was "one" and want to express that way and pull it all in one package, not lock a part of me in a suitcase or desk draw to pull out for amusement or a night out just to be stuffed back in and forgotten like a Christmas or Easter decoration, this was me, my soul and I only have one, I cannot cut it in two pieces and hide it in suitcases and chests, who is who? and the actual feeling of putting yourself away in a draw like that gave me moments of separation anxiety, if that's you in the draw and you have to lock yourself up while the other half walks away to go about life, there is a feeling you are attached to that draw, it's like you put your soul in there, not your "other" identity. And the part walking around is half what it should be, an incomplete person, and I found that very difficult. But at least I felt I had something to identify myself as a woman with, these objects where mine, these little pieces of makeup, jewelry. shoes, clothes, where all little treasures I had at the moment, Instead of an identity I put away in my closet, But I also at times did feel like I was in a battle with two different people one trying to take over and be the one she should be you cannot help that, and we had our own song. Cynthia and I, It was Helen Reddi's you and me against the World. And the makeup and items I had although so easy to obtain by any ordinary girl or woman, who grew into it, for me to go and buy anything, I felt like I was breaking the law, and every camera in the store was on "me", as if I was jacking a car, or stealing, those first two years out there when I come out where terrifying it was so hard to buy my own things, but I calmed down, and that was the key, relaxing into it, if you look nervous people notice, they start to take that second, and that third look, and you feel busted, a warning flag goes up, And now problems arise at work, A new boss! a real micro manager type, at first he seemed ok, but very quiet all the time and just kept to himself, knew little about what any of us did, just talked on the phone to customers all day. Seemed to think everyone he talked to on the phone lie's to him, he said that often, they all lie all of them, and It was getting warm at work summer was coming and a lot of changes in personal where going on, as the company grew and grew, And I was a little concerned, I knew someone there knew and how many I was not sure, I wish I was told who, so I could have relaxed and thought it out more but I was nervous, I did not know what bosses where watching me how high up this went, someone or some people knew I was going to get sex reassignment surgery, when and how, and all the steps and details still unknown to me where going to be found out. Left me in a feeling of suspense, the hormones where really working well my breasts where coming in well. I wore my machine shop coat still to hide them and a sports bra, but it was getting hot, there where high ceilings and cost saving ideas everywhere, one was a regulated temp, and it was hot in a shop jacket, switching to shirts was going to be tricky to keep this private, it was a nice air conditioned cool building but now it's not, shirts had to have pockets the pockets had to have things in them, and a sport bra, with a t-shirt, I had to be careful no one saw the straps, so I wore tank top type t-shirts, under my shirts but you always got those people that love to come up and give you a pat in the back, I was more scared of them than anyone, if anything would give it away it was a pat on the back by the wrong person, paranoia was horrible, I never knew what to expect and kept my back away from people, but the two woman I worked with where always nearby, and there where days I really needed to get down to a T-shirt, a regular T with sleeves, not to look grubby, but those straps even with two light T-shirts where a problem in the heat, I decided to confide in them, At first they thought I was kidding. And when they realized I was not they were excited, happy for me, And excited they had a front row view of a moment only seen on a television show, And they were going to see it in real life and in real time as I went along, they also said that if I had just gone off and did it without telling them they would have been very mad at me, and that I did the right thing coming to them and telling them ahead of time, as by now we were all a little family. But still I had not talked to personal about any steps I was taking. But I was now comfortable at my work area, as months ago by some people notice the changes, I get told by my co-workers someone asked them, I don't pay attention I am so busy working, the workload has almost doubled, we are getting new customers continuously and changing for newer models, keeping up with technology and still producing the older versions to, and they ask questions, is so and so growing breasts,? Or Taking hormones, what's up here, and it is getting back to me, it feels like everyone is starting to take notice, and I take a good look at myself now, and I am developed well a large A-cup but, no doubt the form is nice and perky and I am 37-38 years old and was always in good shape so they really perked right out. They were here, and there was no real hiding them that well anymore, that was proving to be difficult, I talked with my therapist I really wanted a slow quite coming out, my situation involved children, and they have to be considered first The problem with coming out was these programs have is you really make you decide if your strong enough to become a woman and really want it bad enough, You will become a man changing into one right out in the open. And you have absolutely not a private moment to yourself again, everywhere you go. They throw you right into the fire and it burns like hell itself.

And say if you want it that bad this is what you will do to prove it, and it can hurt enough to want to give up and die, it is a real bad approach, I am so glad that there is help now more than when I started twenty years after turning fifteen years old, I was now 35 years old and just put my finger on a doctor in a phone book to start finding help, putting anyone through what they put me through, they may as well have just shot me, you have to go out into it and let everyone watch you slowly change into a woman from a man, and lower yourself from your thrown and become lower than you where before, and a lot of the woman want you to learn the hard way, and you will learn at the bottom of where woman are, they don't think you are good enough to be one of them either, If they know who you are and what you are doing, and god help you if you are a better looking woman than the ones around you, they will not like that at all, and I admit I look good, it is something in my genes or that's just what I am meant to look like, I make a beautiful looking woman, and that helped a lot getting out and around but inside where they all know you, It's a long slow physical and emotional change, that you are put out on a stage for years to be viewed and judged, by people who have no idea of the pain you are already in. before you even decide you need to do this, never mind to go out and display it so publicly, And under the scrutiny of the eye of everyone who is involved in and around your life, be at work, home or the gas station you go to, make mistakes and those that do not accept this will never forget them. The term thrown into the frying pan is a light term, this is the full furnace, and you got to walk along all those hot coals for years to feel like you pass and feel well enough to make it, and changing into a woman in front of everyone with no privacy, You are supposed to want it that bad, that you will be willing to accept all the ridicule, hate and put yourself right in front of those who would murder you and say they did it as favor to the world, is a very dangerous practice used in gender reassignment, there explanation is if you really want to be a woman bad enough you will do it, this is all we got, if you can pass this test you will make it, I tell you I did it, I would again if it's the only way these doctors would let me, but how wrong it is, they will send some out without even starting hormone therapy, just use the clothing and artificial breasts and say be brave, prove it! Prove this is what you want and then we may give you hormone treatments. How wrong and very cruel And how many people have been beaten murdered or lost their jobs from this, and committed suicide, I lost my job, It didn't stop me but I did, the therapist I counted on and needed and spent almost six years of my life with had abandoned me when it got to rough, all I needed was one or two phone calls, Everyone around me at the time I needed them most when I could no longer take this alone, the hate, abuse and discrimination all through the factory I worked in, and left me alone and on my own, was that the test? Did I want it that bad? I did make it, and the doctors who put me and others through that should really know how this is so cruel and barbaric. And at least try and help don't sit back and watch writing it all down for your memoirs, and most likely blame the patient, I got up and on my feet again on my own, I kept going, I was strong enough inside to be this woman I wanted to be, but I don't believe all of us that go through this are, and that's a reason for many suicides, A patient can have a good evaluation from a real gender specialist, even a team of specialists and others who have already gone ahead, Not ever let a person who makes this decision ever have to expose it to anyone at risk of being unessacerally harmed emotionally or physically, no tests or trials outside the doctor's office or clinic to get the hormone treatments he or she needs, the patient if becoming a woman should be feminized and the female to male should be made masculine before attempting to go out there, No change in a workplace, it does not work! Un-less you are lucky and it's a small enough company and everybody is like family and is ok with it, Or changes in laws to protect us and make sure we are safe from abuse, and bullying, it may work well in a company so big you are so lost and no one knows anyone, it is just too big to know every ones business, everyone is just a number type place, then you have a better chance but my first run through was a small factory and everyone knew everyone else's business and the boring work at the assembly lines made making fun of someone something to do for the day to get out quicker, and times when a few moments are confusing to everyone and distracting trouble breaks out and complaints start coming in, It would be nice if an escrow could be set up from each patients account if they wish, As they move forward so money is saved if they don't have it to spend on relocating to a new job and sex reassignment surgery, and insurance is still unwilling to help, these changes I ask for and seek are for young people starting out. Do not ever wait too long to make this decision, get help fast and start as soon as possible, if you get into your twenties it is the beginning of the steep hill you will be building as you wait, and the longer you wait the steeper and the higher the hill will be for you to climb, It should all be kept a secret always, trust few, you will know who, (the patient) should be allowed to do everything he or she needs to do while in the clinical stage, with her or his doctors, With all the changes now and the new understandings from the experiences of those who already went ahead like pioneers I am hoping this book a useful tool for doctor and patient and anyone else in a gender confused state of mind and body, or any person looking to help or understand a friend, or loved one and get the information they need to help them from suffering the regretful consequences of the old idea, of throwing you out into the frying pan, But having and to be giving the knowledge from those that are truly born with crossed genders get the hormones and surgery, and help starting a life they need first. And to adapt with all your new experiences with your emotions because the hardest part of taking hormones out there beginning, is the loss of control of your emotions, I never cried so damn hard as I stepped into that factory every morning to take the abuse I would have to endure, six months after my coming out, and had to watch what started out so well at first, collapse all around me, That was a critical error it was too soon, not as my personality and looks went as much as I was not balanced and adjusted to my hormones and all these stronger emotions, I was not ready, I thought I was, I was an anxious girl waiting to explore, but it was too soon my therapist should have told my company I was not ready, I wanted to hang myself up on the mezzarine where they stored boxes, I wanted to make a little spot behind them like a closet and hang myself off a beam, and the stock boy would have found me, and it came awful close to that, don't try that in a factory like I did, if there is a chance you will be all alone when trouble strikes, then it gets very scary and adjusting to the hormones is no help, move on and away from your past if you need to, If anything is not right anyone in the field as a therapist with real good experience, who knows what to ask will get the right answers back, There are no small differences, an expert in this field can determine the correct patient with talking it out and clinical evaluations, This is "what it's like! approach" I had was very hard and almost killed me, I wonder how many suicides have occurred from this method, and I hope that reading about my life and the struggles I will face, help anyone with their decision to make such a change, do it as early in your life as you can, and have a tool to give themselves careful thought and some of the answers they seek deep inside themselves because that's where we are going, deep inside me, I am a woman, I was born in a male body, I can't tell you how I know, it's a feeling, if you now know then what a rose smells like, I don't have to explain it to you, But if you don't' in this book I am going to become that rose for you. And you will find that there is more to a rose than just its smell alone, you yourself may find you can make a decision that one time so difficult on your own, now hopefully has become an easier decision to make, I want to help! I am to open up and be honest to everyone and be brave and go deep into the roots of my own soul. As far as my heart takes me, take away the sharp edges and thorns so you can hold it right in your own hand, and push through the soft petals to look where I hope you will find some of your own answers, to why and who you are inside! Alone these questions are hard to answer, and we can only sometimes guess and learn from our mistakes, and mistakes don't always give us an answer. but another situation we need to solve, sometimes worse than when we started, it is always good that we can find those who went on ahead of us and where brave enough to test themselves, and to be honest, to the person they most need to love the most, themselves, and share it with those who want or need to follow along. It all started well, I really thought at first a dream come true, after all I followed all the rules, filled in the blanks, dotted the I s at least I thought, there was new management everywhere and personal was all changed a new woman replaced the nurse, she was a regular woman not a nurse a real professional human resource dept. employee. A Very nice woman, but I was curious someone knew, and who was it? Who do I go to update my progress to? Or if I start having co-worker issues, where do I go? My gender therapist was as concerned as I was, my wife and children went, to counseling the two small ones, but the oldest refused, absolutely refused, it was getting close, I was in therapy for years before he saw me dressed as a woman, and I still had little time but I did for practice I joined a social group after his persuading me to join one called tiffany's of new England where all types of transgendered people met to talk and have social events, nothing sexual at all. No alcohol, no smoking. and exclusively private, couple's came, husbands and wives, loner's, the most wonderful most beautiful caring loving people I had ever met in my lifetime, and they are "men", this is where all the good ones are that woman are looking for, I find that these men love there woman and wives so much, they all have long marriage's and all hold hands still, they spend all their time together and they all when not with them, or looking for one to love, or date, say all good things about the woman in their life or the one they hope to find, and my heart went out for many who were afraid like myself to say I am a little different, and are all alone still, I know just how they feel, and there only little flaw is they love to put that little dress on once and a while, they are all good fathers and love their children, so different from the talk I heard in shops and working and garages, a big difference, I was even a hostess many times and loved it, I closed at night, kicked everyone out, cleaned up, got to interview people who wanted to join, I had a place to go, but it was a far ride 90 minutes from my home, so I was tired the next day at work from it. But it was worth it, and only once a week, my therapist and I felt that we had to find who knew what, at work so I could handle anything at this point, and so we knew what to do in any situation, so I went to the woman in personal and introduced myself. I asked if she had heard anything about me that would be unusual or that she felt she needed to know more about at this time, she said no, nothing, nothing? I said back, no nothing! She said, I said ok I will get back to you. This was perplexing, who knew? and it made me nervous, that there was an individual or group of people that knew, and it made me paranoid as hell some days, I knew that the upper people in engineering all meet with the head of the company and the gossip is terrible, I know, as a tool and die maker I knew them all well and was in those meetings to discuss how to build tooling, Not all of them because I was so busy, but there where days I could not help feel alerted, who are they? I loved factory work and the people, we had a lot of Vietnamese and Hatiane people, I worked with them all and helped a lot of them read and right our language, The company had a teacher come in and they had a class, but I gave them the extra they needed out on the floor, when they got stuck on their progress reports and work sheets, and it made it easier for me as I interact with so many of them that the learning our language was a plus for both, and I had made a lot of friends, Some of the Vietnamese who are great martial artists return home to fight for the family honor, in friendly but fierce competitions they are skeptical about Americans. Or the quay Lounge (round eye) but even they would trust me to ask them to check their spelling and there sentence structure, they were all wonderful people and one lead Vietnamese man I would befriend I would have reading and writing English like a pro, this guy was getting a Boston accent, I had become so close as friends he said he was taking me to Vietnam to raise hell with him, I knew a day was coming he was to know this male American friend, he has found and has had such a good relationship with, was going to change into a woman, and telling him I found the hardest part inside the company I would have to do, There was one other man, a very kind looking guy had a harmless look with those Clark Kent glasses very quiet, kept to himself, Came to me one day out of the blue and said, how far along are you, I said with what? I got scared, he said! Martial arts! I thought something else, and was so relieved. I thought he had figured me out and read me. I said how did you know? He said it's in you. it's all over your character, the way you walk, move, watch and observe people, when I see you in a room I know that if attacked you can handle yourself, he said he has trained his whole life, he was lucky to find an old Asian gentlemen living in his neighborhood, who he had worked hard for many years doing yard work, like painting, helping him take care of his home for free, He was a kid with nowhere to go, took years before he would he even speak to him. He just watched, and I am not saying it was anything like the movie karate kid, he had it easy, and this was reality. He gave him lessons in an art of meditation that along with the right exercises can give him the strength to punch right through a brick wall with his hand, And he was not lying he demonstrated some of his skills and taught me the firsts steps of building the force of my chi and how to use it to add strength to what I already have, Meditation of a type I had not known but when shown made so much sense, I share it with no one and keep it to myself, He became such a close friend at the end of my employment there, And the day when I made my appearance this powerful man I had met, He was probably one of the most dangerous people out walking the streets of New England, with his hands and skills alone, would leave "me" A note! at my bench my first day I come in as Cynthia, that reads I admire your courage, even I don't have that much, and that meant a lot to me, it helped then and it still helps me to this day, he did a lot for me with that little note, I wish he would come across my book and read this, I wish him well I hope his life has gone on and he is where he wants to be right now, and how funny to me. how far I am going to go into womanhood, and how far I am taken myself away from the warrior male I was becoming, you know a real truthful warrior, he is one who's word is most sacred to himself, when he tells you he has given his word he will not harm you, he will not!, not ever, the pseudo warrior males word is not sacred to himself or anyone, he will tell you, you are safe to go but later, harm you. Those are, the differences that define the two, in my life time I was very close to the feel of what it means to have the skills and strength and courage to fight and protect myself and my loved ones without hesitating, were in the generation I live in now I would not have been considered a warrior but if I was born one hundred fifty years ago as a male with these skills on a reservation, under the same circumstances I would have been a great warrior and have succeeded there also, and I know I would have had all the same results, in the end, and in this book about sex change I am hoping to help distinguish the fetish and fantasy from the real feeling of being a woman and not just a cross dresser. That most people even yourself might think you are, so my therapist and I decide we move forward. A time to be "me" is approaching, And it is decided no harm in telling the woman in personal where I am going, she is told and surprised, not anything she would have thought, And I told her I would update her on the changes as I went along. And told her I felt some employees new, they may have noticed or heard rumors, and that I had told my two co-working females, I now had to decide on a name, I hadn't given that much thought yet, but it was time. My wife called me Angela; she said I changed to such like an angelic person in that persona. That she liked it and where I took her from a family she did not ever feel a lot of affection from, as if it I was angel came and rescued her. I did not want that permanent, as nice as it was and she liked it. It was not so much the changing into the clothing that made me like that, it was I was so more relaxed in them and I felt like somebody finally liked "me", and was not scared by my gentle touch but enjoyed it, "there are woman" who do, but the name Angela it was to coined, to many cross dressers had that name along with Tina, Tiffany, Angel, Terry, I needed a strong female name but very feminine. I looked at a book, with names for babies it had to be sensible and right like I wanted to be "right. I found Cynthia and read the meaning of what it meant.

It was the Greek goddess of the moon. And also the flower the Chrysanthemum was another name for Cynthia. It was perfect. I loved it, and what about a middle name, I thought Cynthia sue, Ann, Lou, back to Ann Marie sounded close but to long Marie, Marie fit, it rolled nice, it was familiar to, and I wrote it down to look at it, Cynthia Marie, yes! That's me! I said loud inside I added my last name put it in my pocket and went to the court house to file for a change of name, also which because I was married had to get a release signed by my spouse that it was ok. And I got it. And I was going to change it and keep it private for a while; Massachusetts has its own special common law name laws. I could legally be Cynthia and still keep my male name till I was ready to come out all the way, I went to the clerk and told them I was here to petition for a name change, and he said what do you want to change your last name to? I said not my last, my first, he said well that is unusual ok, I handed my paperwork and fee and when he looked he just looked back and just grinned at me, not to be nice either, I left and waited for the court to summon me into a hearing to explain why I wanted to change my name. I got the needed paperwork from my gender therapist, and went into court, a woman judge calls me to the bench leans over and whispers, is this name change for a sex change? I said yes, she said, well normally we need some sort of paper work and proof you are really what you say you are, and you have doctors and not just doing this on your own, and this is not a mistake you will regret later, I said ok and handed her what paper work my therapist gave me, she looked them over quick and said I will give you my answer in several weeks also first you will receive a document with your change of name request, you have to go to the town newspaper you live in and show it to them to prove you are legally changing your name, And doing so in public so as not to hide from any crimes or tax or debts you may still owe and be held accountable to. Once that is done show a receipt from the newspaper company, proving to us you have and complied with the court and everything will move forward and I will make my decision, so it comes. And I go to the newspaper and tell them I am changing my name and that it needs to be in the paper, I ask they make it personal as possible being the sensitive subject it is, they say ok, but we need this record of proof you are changing your name to go ahead and we will mail it back to you. It will be in next month's paper we only deliver every month and all seems ok. I can ride it out, I feel good I am changing, the feeling of coming to life is approaching and about to knock at the door, now there are physical and legal changes, my name will be a woman's name soon. I feel attached to myself. I have time I can take a year or two to prepare for the worst of what could be, and take my time getting ready, But not to be so, it would be a month instead of years, the newspaper instead of being discreet took the entire court document and blew it up to take an entire page of the newspaper, a very private moment of my life was suddenly all over town, when I went to get the newspaper myself to see the article. I am horrified at what I see, I cannot believe they did that to me, as if they played a cruel joke, and now I had to go and tell my oldest daughter real fast, like in minutes, before it broke out all over town and she heard from her friends, this was a nightmare. it was the worst thing that could have happened with this name change, it had my address and everything, some nut could have shot me coming out my front door claiming he did the world a favor, And this day was the beginning of hell, that I would endure for three years from my oldest daughter till she is removed from the home, and another 17 years till I have to finally say goodbye for good, as she cannot accept Cynthia, she wants her dad back and that's it! Nothing else, telling her was one of the hardest things I ever did as if I had died and my spirit had enough energy to come and tell her. I will never forget that moment as long as I live, and it was all too soon and so un-nessacary but for some foolish people looking for sensationalism working for their boring town newspaper, they made me put a hurt into my little girl she and I were just not ready for, She may never have been ready, but the way it just blew around town like that, was the worst nightmare of how it could have happened, the night I told my daughter her dad was becoming a woman. I never saw her cry so hard, it did not seem like she was ever going to stop, and time for a while just stood still. I wanted to die a lot more than she did, I know that, I wanted to die a lot more than anyone would ever know, when you can say something to who, was once a beautiful baby of your own in your own arms and hurt it so bad, life just loses its feeling of what it means, It took me months to recover the grief I felt, I only hoped she found some strength to realize how much of inside of myself hurt so much that it had come to make a change in my life like this to finally be happy, but she never did. It was forever a struggle and with knowing that she would never accept me I was still as determined as ever to move forward, I had come this far, And I was always going to give love a chance to grow, always gave out love, sometimes that small little seedling will get its nourishment and come out of the ground all anew sometimes they wither and dry out and die, I am still hoping the rays of the sun will come through someday, but

hope is running away as my lifetime runs away with it. I need to grow also. And I will. I push myself through the many weeds of the garden I was planted in and I survive, and I am finding the hormones physical effects and the upcoming change in my name uplifting in spirit but my oldest daughter and her boyfriend are still explosive, police seem to know us to well and he is finally going, he is packed ready to go. But again stays, I want a restraining order but I need my wife in with me, she owns the apartment to, but I find her reluctant, she seems to like this guy, they have befriended each other, she is not as willing to get the order some out of fear of retaliation from her daughter, she has been hit very hard before, she told years later when I went to work, my oldest daughter would enter the room and say I am in charge now you will do what I say, to her mother, and I was never told, And I know that this will be a very hard thing to deal with, Soon I am approached at work by the woman from personal she said they had talked to their company doctor who recommends they get a consultant to help move the company with the transition, she would come in while I took a long week end off and train the employees in gender reassignment in the workplace And that the management would go first before employees, and I would get to meet with her first, This sounded great, they seem to want to help, and I said that would be ok. And I informed my therapist who also said great, this is wonderful. And we "all" agreed that open communications between all of us would be important and nessacary to make this work, it all seemed to make things go faster than I was prepared at home for, My wife began to back down and seemed like this is not what she put in for, but I told her the company has done a lot of work and they want to move forward, it will be ok, I have a job, the kids are seeing a counselor if they need to and we will go slow, the plan is that I must wear a dress the first 6 months everyday no matter what, the reason is recognition as a woman, It is important and a dress symbolizes a woman and people will perceive you as a woman quicker and easier, so it's good you keep in that type of clothing. And that is fine with me, not at home, my wife wants a slower approach for the kids and the neighbors are going to be hard on us for this, I feel she is right, and I do my best always to compromise, I never did any of this selfishly for my own need, I always thought of everyone around me especially the children and my two youngest, my middle one is the sweetest of all. I never even have to scold her I spanked her once when she was fresh to her mother

just a tap, She was so embarrassed and hurt she got red all over her face, I never could again and she never needed to be disciplined ever again not even to be scolded, she was that good and still is, and is the only child I have that I feel I can talk about anything to, I almost lost her, she almost drown in a fish tank, it was down low, I had two, one on top and one on the bottom shelf of the cabinet, it was an old television console, I took the television out and put a fish tank inside and one on top, it had doors to shut it so something like that would not happen, but when they were little they swung on them and broke them off. she climbed into her little sisters walker, and was too big for it and tipped over, Her head popped right through the middle of a 25 gallon tall fish tank, lucky I was right there ironing I saw her tip over and hear a loud pop, and she is stuck inside the tank, water is just trickling out around her neck, I ran and lifted her as straight as I could and pulled her out, she was like a cork, when I pulled her out twenty five gallons of water filled up the downstairs real fast, it is a lot of water when it's dumped all of a sudden, I had no time to check wires and plugs I ran to the couch as fast as I could, and lay her down expecting the worse, I even thought she may be dead, Not a scratch on her, she hit it just right and popped through the glass, But I know if I was not there and acted quick and she tried to get herself out she may have almost severed her head from the loose glass hanging like a guillotine, I was never so scared in my life as I was that moment, I never put a tank low again ever, And getting through work and keeping my job is important to make a living to take care of my children and also, for sex reassignment surgery you must have full time employment. Or a way to have an income that is permanent to satisfy the surgeon to get surgery, They don't want to do all that then leave you out there with no income and homeless, they think of that at least and that is more the surgeon who I find is more concerned about that, that it is his priority that I am ok to support myself out there and not be alone, and penniless, so many have ended up that way, nowhere to go and no one to love them, They die out on the streets all alone, and no one cares. They get a better funeral from strangers than the people that once loved them or where family, I personally love the idea I am finally in my life coming to work in a dress, This to me is amazing, if anyone is in the program "I am" I start buying dresses and I also buy a nice long coat a nice long black cotton p-coat style 'all the way down to my feet to help hide what I wear for the kids, though the shoes always, and the bottom of some skirts show, I move ahead I take my long weekend and get ready for what I expect to be a scary and also what I want at the same time fun, like in line for the scary roller coaster ride you have always feared but wanted to ride so bad, and now it's time to sit down strap in and hang on, So in I go, I leave early, I always did but we were having a snow storm and I left extra early, I wanted to beat everyone to work, that was the plan, and guess what? I get a flat? Right on the highway, And if I wait for anyone to help it will be hours and I will be on the news, as the car that broke down causing all the trouble that morning, so what do I do? I get out and fix my flat tire myself, on a 1978 Fleetwood Cadillac, cars everywhere, out there in a snowstorm, on the highway, in a dress, lucky I had gloves, or I would have ruined my nails, and had a spare, people honked their horns at me, swore at me, move that f' ing car lady What.! But I did it, and was so glad I was called a lady, I never changed a tire so fast in my life, I got into work and made it early and it all went great, I got a real good reception one that would last for several months then turn completely upside down, and bring an end to my almost six year employment, In the meantime, work was very busy, and a woman I worked with was very friendly very young and was very curious about this man working beside her with a dress on, makeup, heels, the whole nine yards they call it, therapists call it, out in full gear. It intrigued her, she was more than just curios in a why do you? As in more I would love to sleep with someone like you just to see what it's like. She said it's as close to being with a woman as she can get without really being with one, so there would be no quilt feeling that she slept with one, I told her I was flattered that she even considered me as a sex partner either way, or in any romantic encounter, but that I was married and that I never have cheated on my wife, and that this would only make things at work more difficult and the no! was taken to heart, she got mad, I rejected her and she would not talk to me, and this would repeat itself many times over the course I was there till she finally left, and she was very pretty and any guy would take her out, but just like with my wife, I was not in this for the sex, I was in this for my soul, But it became an annoyance to my boss who noticed we were not getting along, and I was talking to my therapist and some people in personal about what to do And what sexual harassment meant and how do I define this problem, this was so unexpected, she was so curios, I never thought that would happen, how do I tell anyone and do it all without dropping a name? I needed an out from this, and work was as crazy as it gets. I was doing the work of two people, some days three, I was keeping up but there were some loose ends, I could not complete every part of a job. I worked an eight hour day five days a week, I needed more time and hours but was not able to get them, and then a boy in the stockroom kept calling me sir! And was impolite, the employees all had a class and all were told not to do things like that, but he did, and not every time, just a jab here and there, when I went and got a part I needed from stock. He would put in that little jab, ok sir! Thank you sir! So I went to a head of the human resource's dept. I knew well and told him about it, and asked him that he not punish anyone, as it would have a negative effect, just go and have a man to man talk and let him know that people need to be treated with respect, no matter who or what they are, and he agreed, Two days later I am about to leave my area and his coworkers on a large fork truck blocked the door way and just glared at me, it was a standoff? No! not for me, I just put my hands together at my tummy and put my head down And waited for them to leave, they suddenly looked ashamed of themselves and backed away, but that was the beginning of the trouble, it went out I was a rat and got him in trouble, which I did not do, he was just told not to be so impolite to anyone, no written warning nothing just told be more polite, even the two woman I worked with took his side, they said I should have just gone to his supervisor and not so high up. But I did not know who his supervisor was, they were all just young stock room boys I thought they were all the same level just maybe one was there longer than the rest, soon we had a bring your kids to work day! and I asked my two youngest daughters to come and they said they would, I was so happy, I hoped everyone would see I was a nice family person with nice kids, And that day was good, it brought down some barriers, And some woman who would not ever talk to me before, soon did, It started to go back to normal. But the work load kept piling up and piling up. I was now getting all the new products and was responsible to make sure that they sealed right, a gasket sat inside the switches we made, and a press pushed the top on and a die rolled over the edges to hold it together and make it water tight and that the height of the complete switch had to be within a few thousands of an inch, to get the correct travel and get the voltage reading at a measured out length that meant it was assembled correctly. And there where many other intricate measurements to each switch to pass inspection and to record into a book and chart the progress but the setup for the compression was a long process and with the newer lines along with the older ones also left no time to fill the spc chats for quality control and also I put the switches on a test machine that made them work ten years' time In two days, then look for defects, that I did, not one product of mine ever came back, But my boss was losing his mind over the charts, sitting there putting in the numbers and connecting a series of dots to get a graph, It is easy but not when there is no time to do it, Customers come into look at those graphs to check the quality awareness of the company, I needed two more of me to do all the work, the others were lying in their books they just copied what was there and fudged it, there products where different they could, they came off automated machines that gave them print outs, mine did not, I had to do all mine by hand, and I fell behind, I was getting called into the office daily even though there products came back rejected, I get yelled at two or three times a day and along with my co-worker that still was making her attempts to sleep with me and was getting turned down, and was getting him mad because we weren't getting along, and he didn't know the real reason yet but he said get along and work together, one day after finally getting what information I needed and felt I had enough of this girls pranks, She did some mean things to me, I thought I could confide in her, but everything I told her she went around and told everyone else, all over the plant, real personal things, girl talk things, I thought I had a girlfriend to talk about things and learn from, but she gave me the opposite advise, just to hurt me, once we had a picnic at the company and I told her I would like to sit and see if anyone will come and sit with me and not be shy or afraid of me, but she told a group of them what I was doing and as a joke don't sit over there with her, I looked up and saw her with everyone laughing, but the good thing was all the bosses and higher ups sat with me instead so it didn't work out as she hoped but that was some of the mean things she did, and the other woman I worked with would bang the toilet seat down three times real hard to warn everyone I was coming so they could all get out real fast as if I was coming in for a peep show, they were rebelling I was using the ladies room, I had a handicap bathroom key, but when I felt ready I could switch, but after I did and saw the discrimination and fear I asked for my key back, they said no, you can't go backwards, I went into my boss finally and said we need to talk I have a serious problem

with a certain co-worker, And he just looked at me and said I don't
care! I am not interested in any problems you are having with who you
work with just go do your job, I was shocked, I had nowhere to go and
I did not know where to take it from here except to go way over his head
way over, and that meant real hard feelings but it was coming, and then
something good happens real good, I win 100,000,.00 in a lottery
drawing, And I receive 67,000.00 after taxes, I have vacation time so I
plan to take two weeks off in October and take my entire family to
Florida, "Disney Land" first time in my life I get to go there and my
kids are at a good age, the bad part I don't like, is my oldest daughter
without asking me invites her boyfriend, I was very upset, they were
just about to break up, I was working late, I could not leave work and
asked my wife to play my numbers for me, and gave her my numbers I
wanted played, and that morning went to work, when I hear the number
at first I am surprised I said no way, and then I remember my wife was
going to play it for me. I call to check and try to be calm, she said yes I
did play it, I said tell me the numbers you played for me, and she reads
them off and says why what's up did you win? I said I am not sure yet I
may have but I want to look at the ticket myself before I believe it, keep
it in your room, lock it up in the safe and whatever you do not tell
anyone especially our oldest daughter's boyfriend they are breaking up,
let it happen. If he knows we have money like that we will never get rid
of him, and she promises me she won't, I tell my boss I think I won
some big money and to my surprise he seemed happy about it, He said
leave early if you want, go find out, so I leave, and there is my wife
squeezing the life out of the ticket it was so wet from sweat it was
almost no good, and guess who is the first congratulating me,? him, My
daughter's boyfriend, she ran right in and told him, and at first refused
to let me see the ticket, her true nature came right out, she said it's mine
all of it, I won this money, I played it, I am the winner every penny is
mine, and I say look you, it's not all yours I picked those numbers, I
won! and look at yourself, your forgetting your even married, you
should be ashamed of the way you are acting, give me my ticket, let go
of it, and she handed it to me, she did but that moment I really learned
a lot about her, she was a selfish woman always was, and so is my first
daughter who she raised, but this time it really showed, I looked at my
ticket, I won, it was soaked in sweat, I did not even know if the machine
would pick up the bar code, And to top it off that monster of a boyfriend

Cynthia Marie

was all up in there going we are rich we are rich, like he won, like he was a family member, he had by then unpacked all his stuff and was there to stay, that was the worst part about the timing of winning that money, if I wasn't so damn busy and played it myself I would have kept quiet till he left. And was sure he was out of our lives before I told anyone, But all that was ruined and my daughter was to suffer another 2 years of beatings and abuse and get left with his child, that I would eventually end up raising, till he was 14 years old and till I finally just made his mother take him back, I asked my wife's father to put it in an account for us to protect it and where he was over the age of 65 it would be tax free. and that he could keep the 33,000 The government took out for taxes for himself, but he declined, and would regret it later he did not help his daughter, My name is all changed now and we are all set to go to Florida, All that happened that last January when I got all my court documents and went to social security and the registry, there was about a month I had to use my old name at work, cashing my check the first time at the bank was very funny, The girl thought it was me but was not sure what to do, but decided to cash it, then after that everything went smoother, once a salesman who came to our house weekly to get payments for furniture was in line at the bank, I just noticed him as he was just looking at me and I turned real quick, I don't know if he saw me or not, he never said anything but had a silly grin the next time I saw him, all the restaurants and gas stations I went to who knew me before, where just shocked, at first, and a lot said so who put you up to this,? Lose a bet with someone? I got a lot of that, but at least they all complimented me, they all said I looked great, they would never have known, and that gave me a lot of confidence, things changed so much, whistles from cars, guy's pulling up beside me honking and hanging out the windows, it was awesome that I got the attention like that, But also it was new to me I had forgot that I would attract men, and I never expected I would get such good results, I was a man magnet it seemed odd and funny at times and took a long time to get used to getting doors opened for me, in fact now I notice if I hold a door open for someone especially a woman she really looks real close at me, Because I shouldn't be doing it, old manners, even polite ones I have to break are giveaways, and things like that are one of them, I was passing and doing well. With men anyway, woman, they were harder at first, I only passed less than 50 percent of the time, this had to change, they were all nice but they all

120

gave that little I know what you are smile and I wanted to be perfect and had to perfect myself to pass woman as a woman and once I reach that point I would start to get more comfortable, It was like a thermometer, watching the gage go up each year as I got better at makeup and the hormones really started to make changes all over that you don't think they do, but even the shape of my eyes would change, so when people get close and look at me in the eye they are looking at woman's eyes, and that is a big help up close especially when I have to approach woman, Our trip to Disney land was great but my wife wanted to stay with her sister. who now lived down near Miami I did not want to stay there at all, I wanted to do the whole resort thing and go all out, but she really wanted to be with her sister for a day or two and I said ok, as long as they are nice to us we can stay, after all, we are bringing our daughter's boyfriend and to me it just took the family experience out of it. It changed everything and to make it worse, the two fought the whole time we were there, I almost sent them home on an airplane early just to get rid of them, they ruined a great experience, and why my wife ever agreed to this is beyond me, I said no, I did not want to bring this guy he was trouble, always was and always will be. and I knew he would ruin our stay down there and he did, he put rain in where there should have been nice sunny days, but there was a part of me that was afraid of him being there without us up in our hometown, he was a thief, he may have come back to our apartment while we were gone and broke in, I had a lot to think about all the time, I was always stressed out, and the first night we arrive in Florida, I am exhausted I had to work that day, drive everyone to the airport, and get the rental and drive to my wife's sisters house where we are met with so much inhospitality I was shocked, We could not even breath without them looking at us, they assumed because we were with a black guy we had all kind of drugs on us or something, her sister kept saying no pot in my home no way not even in my yard, nowhere, and this woman one time was a drug dealer sold coke, crack, pot, LSD, you name it she did it and sold it, and now she is telling us she has been born again, and none of that will be tolerated in her Christian home. After her long boring full of bologna speech, I just went to bed I did not care about things like that I just wanted to sleep and at the worst I might want to do is smoke some pot before I go to Disney Land, but that's about it, and it's so funny to me that she would say all this then drink down a gallon of cheap wine, She is a big woman and she can handle a gallon, and she sure did, that night, and that morning I had to face her hung over and with a surprise I get that I did not know was coming, But she got nosey or was just out looking for something in our car we rented, and as I am having a cup of coffee trying to wake up from a horrible sleep, them partying real loud on booze. And in the morning the sprinklers came on. and the smell of the water that they use in Florida for watering your lawn is the foulest smelling water I ever had to smell my entire life, only one time on Nantasket beach Massachusetts after many, many northeaster's the seaweed and dead animals and fish of the sea piled up for months rotting away in the sun had I ever smelled something again that would make want to vomit, I had to wake up to that and another nightmare, as I sit there half-awake drinking coffee, my wife's sister is flipping through papers, I thought just her mail or fliers, I had no idea she had gone out to the rental car and took the paper work out with the rental agreement and insurance information, And looks up at me right in the eye and real loud says, who is Cynthia Marie? You could hear a pin drop. I was stunned! everyone all of a sudden looked at me, everyone, like I had the answer, but I kept quiet I looked at my wife for a clue or a hint to come here, talk quick, but nothing just silence and a room full of people just staring at me, except my wife, She was looking at the floor, and not saying a word, and again she says ok you guys! Who is this Cynthia Marie? I am reading it right here! someone in this room explain to me, who this is, I want to know right now, who Cynthia is, so I say it's me, she just stares at me and says you? You're Cynthia? Yes I am! Why? So what's the story to this? Why are you calling yourself Cynthia? And by now I am alone here, everyone I came with is still just staring, and her family, her three boys and husband all just there staring. If someone could just give me a quick line, an excuse something, I am half a sleep and getting questioned by a hung over angry 350 lb. woman and I just don't know what to say but the truth, I am tired and I have had a lot of stress to get this far. For the first time in years I am on a vacation, and this woman is not interfering with that, and I just out right tell her, I have decided to become a woman, I am in a sex reassignment program and that is my legal name now and I am legally a female I took out my license showed it to her it had all the correct information name dob and sex. Markers "F" no more "M" and she just tapped her feet and said nothing just tapped her feet. I got up from the table went into my room.

Got all my stuff, packed it up, and said I am leaving, you can stay here but not me I am finding a place to go stay, this is horrible how they are treating me and all of us, so we just left, and we found a nice resort to stay at, we later met with them and bought them tickets too Disney land and I hope it would be better now and they were going to at least be friendly but no they just shied away, did not talk to me much, did not appreciate the tickets I bought for them at 120 dollars apiece an all-day go anywhere pass, they just said we come here all the time, this is just another weekend for us, They had money it was nothing to them, just a normal weekend., Except for meeting Cynthia, When we left Florida, on the flight home my daughter's boyfriend cries, He is scared of flying and he has real tears this time, the way down he just chewed his nails and slept, not this time, a stewardess has to comfort him, and he takes a tranquilizer, I am so surprised, He acts like such a hoodlum and a street tough guy why is he crying,? And his name is so Arabic If it was post 911 they would have brought the airplane down to see what he was really doing. Two weeks later her sister would fly up from Florida and visit each of her family members to tell them my personal business and that she would tell them all she would spend her last penny and last dying breath to break My marriage apart, what hurt most was the very close relationship I had with my mother in law, she was so envious of, my wife's mother did not like her other daughters husband, she knew he was so corrupt and had corrupted her daughter when they were teens, she liked me, I drove her home from the parties when she had too much to drink instead of her husband, I could wave from the window to her, but never could I come in to give her a hug again and tell her hello. And she replaced my mother, she was like my new mother, I really was close to her, I never get to feel close to anyone, I know I scare everyone away, She had a few years earlier a massive stroke that left her partially paralyzed and after that, The father shut the door on us all, I felt like I did when I lost my first friend from kindergarten "Mary Lou" when her mother said I shouldn't play with girls anymore, And could only wave at the window, it was the same thing, same feeling, only I am so much older now, and it hurt a lot more now than then, I understood more this time, there would be no more social gatherings there any longer. Another home gone, he took over, even my wife got very few visits, and by appointment only, most he would cancel. We always felt if we got to see her more and got her active she would have recovered a lot better and lived a happier life and had more fun, than just being handed a remote for the television and a frozen dinner, But for a while at least I got in once in a while for a hug, but after her sister came up from Florida, the door was slammed in my face, and that's just what I mean, I stopped to visit one day about a few months after she had made her trip from Florida and her vow to destroy me, and our marriage to see if it was safe to just visit and say hello, and try to maybe get one more hug before she passed on And I could tell her or explain myself and say my side and not what a revengeful child has come to report to their parents, And that's what I got, the door slammed in my face, by her husband we are too busy to see 'YOU'! I just waved bye at the window, and she waved back, Just like my old first friend Mary Lou. And the Sad part for me also was her name was Mary too, she looked so sad, but there was nothing she or I could do, she looked like a prisoner to me by a control freak male who has finally got the control he always wanted, and to make it even worse, my three children go to visit their grandmother on Christmas day with gifts in their arms, smiles on their faces, and a door slammed in their faces too. My own children his granddaughters, the only ones he has, the rest are grandsons five of them. My daughter was his first grandchild, but he says his grandson from his oldest son is, and we got him beat by two years, and he slams a door in there face on Christmas day itself December 25th. A day to forgive cherishes and love, a day I or my daughters will never forget for the rest of there or my life. How cruel was that. They all cried so hard that day, and now as I write this book the father has now passed on and the two brothers brought over a couple of chairs, this entire time I have written this book I have sat in the chair once Mary my mother in law sat in by the window when I waved to her, it is now my chair I started in November of 2011 it's now February 2012 as I redo and edit this book, this now being the 20th Feb, I have gotten to my tenth draft of the book I gave out the eigth to some close friends for feedback, and I hope if they liked it and get to this part in the new draft I hope my final, that they see this and know how much I appreciate them and love them all for understanding me and just being a kind generous friend, I never in my life wrote a book or never thought to much about it or really read a pile, of them, I took out all the names as many as possible to protect myself and friends, but I find one name that repeats and it was at first by accident but now so important to me, the name is Mary, my first friend from kindergarten I played as a girl with till she was taken, then my mother in law Mary I was close to the door slammed in my face and the third, Mary, the mother of god, when I reach that time in my life will the door be slammed once more, or will I get my wish and be taken in and embraced as a woman in heaven, it is what I so patiently await as my time grows so close now, and this man's hate is so sudden and extreme I respected him his entire life and took care of his daughter and granddaughters, who he now refuses to even acknowledge, and also he had a gay son, one he had spent about a hundred grand on keeping him out of trouble and buying cars he smashed that insurance wouldn't cover, because he was stoned drunk all the time. Helped him buy a home with a gay lover helped him completely gut out the house and redo it, even dug out the dirt floor for a basement. All that was ok till near the end when his son pushed a little too far, and when he found out he was dying from cancer of the bladder and it had spread to the kidney, He asked for his share of a trust fund, he wanted his money before he died, his father said no! You do not want it for yourself you want to die and leave it for your male lover! I am not giving you another dime, and he meant it and a big firestorm in the family ignited, he was shut out like me, the door was slammed in his face too, Not a penny to him not even for his life saving medicines and pain medicine that he had become addicted too, from an injury he had as a teenager in an automobile accident trying to commit suicide, He almost lost a leg, it looked terrible, like a shark bit his calf right off, on his left leg his family treated him terribly at the end and said he was nothing but a sinning homosexual drug addict and was evil, and had become possessed by the devil and he only wanted the money for male whores, And drugs and to satisfy the needs of his young male lover, But it was not true, He was dying, I took him to the hospital where he had his tests done and I read all his medical reports, I was a medical assistant and knew how to read medical reports, It was sad, I knew just how he felt, his family just suddenly throwing him out into the cold, and I get a call, one day a few months after I had taken him into the hospital for his tests, he is dead, but not from the cancer, he was doing laundry and when he went up the stairs, Slipped out of a loose slipper fell down backwards, and broke his neck, His boyfriend found him, and the family had the police grill him, They said he probably killed him for his money but he is cleared, and also one day just after the death, they broke in to get their hands on his will so he would not be able to leave his male lover anything. especially the house the father put all that money into, but they were too late, and also the safe had the fathers, fathers, fathers, solid gold watch worth 50,000 at least, what a beauty, and it was gone, he took it all out before they ransacked the house, he got the last laugh on them, He was expecting them to do that, it was half his home, he could have had them all arrested, But my brother in law to me was murdered by hate. More than just a loose slipper took him from here, a long history of hate and abuse and drugs, and his family telling him what a sinner he was, and when he needed them only offered a prayer instead of a good deed, all of them have a lot of money and are very well off, but the way they are brought up is they are only for themselves they would let my wife their own sister die starving in the street and if they saw her collapse would be more concerned they might miss their bus rather than stop to see if she is ok, that's just the way that Father was and how he brought them up, I pray for them all the time that they will change and live by what they keep saying, about their strong faith in god and how they are so concerned for every ones soul, but I see nothing change in the months after my wife's Fathers death, they rarely talk to her though they promised they would, and treat her like a child, and are holding back on giving her own trust fund as long as they can, I have been brutally harassed myself and one thing that happens under that type of stress, is you get very weak, Especially in your legs, and they shake, even walking is very difficult when you are beating down so emotionally by cruel people, who think what you are doing is selfish and perverted, the exact opposite of what you really are, going upstairs is very hard, and he had one bad leg already, he also told me if he could find a way to kill himself and could make it look like an accident, he would, and if he got real bad news and felt that he would be able to leave his lover money to move on he would, And that he said he wanted to leave his siblings money but they had been so awful to him in the last months of his life that he in no way would, But also he knew his lover had another, and was beginning to suspect it was more than just plutonic, and was starting to find out they may be trying to adopt a child without him knowing, but an agency called several times and he was suspicious and was thinking of taking him out of some of his wills and leaving some to my wife, and his nieces, not me, just them, we got along good He was a very intelligent man to talk to, and very educated. He did hit on me once, but I told him, I am like your sisters wife it would be like being with your sister, almost incest, so stop and think about that, and he did he said your right, I never thought of it like that, but his lover hated me and did not want me to even call the house, he said I was a tease? And I liked to look like that to turn gay men on then reject them, it was the first time I ever heard that one, with a man's version There are so many double standards in life, but I did any way, I was the only one in the family that helped him the last months of his life get what he needed and got him where he needed to go, My wife and her brother that died where close, but he died before he could change anything, His funeral was one of saddest things I ever saw, only the dad, His two brothers, a sister two sister in laws and my wife and I, have a funeral, they open the ground with the back end of a shovel, barley six inches deep if that, about three or four feet long and just dump his ashes right in, Cover him up and walk away, as if he never existed, and that's what they say at the end of it all and to this day that he is gone we need to forget him, they don't even tell people they meet new in their lives they had a brother that died, he is gone and forgotten, I went to visit his grave months ago and I can't even find it, there is no plaque stone or any remains that indicate a body is buried under all the bushes that have over grown in the garden, someday when they need to remove plants in the future what will happen to his remains, are they thrown into a compost heap, What an end, I think about mine now, because of his and I know now I better plan for it, Now!! I do not want to end like him thrown out and forgotten, and the people that knew me and really loved me, not knowing I was ever gone, and have a chance to say goodbye somewhere, somehow in their own way, but they can't, if they never find out. It was early November and we are back from Florida and work is horrible now. Every day I am getting called into my bosses office and told I am not doing my job, I am just doing things I like to do and that I am taking advantage of the companies generosity by thinking I can get away with doing anything I want, because I think I am special, I am so shocked, I said that is so untrue, I appreciate everything this company has done for me, and I need a job to complete all this, a job is important to me more than even to you, how can even say anything like that to me at a time like this, and with the emotional stress that you yourself know I have to deal with out there, I am really trying, you have given me the work of three people, But he just laughs it off, I say are you planning on firing me? Because you've already had me sign warnings, I feel I may be getting systematically fired, you are just following the procedures your mind is made up, and he said, yes! I am going to fire you! not now, it takes time, but I am going to fire you, after that every day I am yelled at blamed and humiliated daily Several times a day, tears run from my eyes all day long just an endless streams of tears everyone sees it, but pays no mind it's as if I asked for it. And my requests for transfers are denied, less qualified are giving jobs I could do. Injuries or not I could still do these jobs I applied for, I had to get away from this dept. this boss, but no nothing, they say what are you going to move away from? everyone is still here, and I suspect while in Florida my two co-workers said anything they could to discredit me, by then we were barely talking, and it was childish of them, I was in so much pain, and they knew it I cried in front of them and they just laughed it off, they do not understand it is just this one area that is a problem that affects me everywhere else but I cannot get through to them, I ask my therapist to call my employer and try to help me with this somehow, He tells me there company doctor has to call him first, so I go and I tell them, and they tell me there doctor said the same thing, that my doctor has to call their doctor first, and I have paid my therapist good money I really felt he should call but after asking once more he said no, it's not the way he would do it, It would be unprofessional of him to approach, I feel myself he wants to be paid by my company for a phone consultation, And that is where the problem is, but it should not! Two doctors to exchange information when release papers have been signed should be just that pick a phone up and call, it is too much, I never could to this day figure out why at that moment he pulled away I felt abandoned, It's now thanksgiving time it just breaks I can no longer take it.

It's the 22nd and the anniversary of JFK'S assassination a very sad day in my memory, like many of us who lived through that, so I was not cheerful I never am on that day, As a child I cried with the nation as I watched over and over the television of news reports and saw Kennedy playing like a dad with his children. People all over the world cried, the whole world seemed to stop and cry that thanksgiving weekend in 1963, a dad was shot dead, gone, taking from his family I went into personal and said good bye I cannot take this, you cannot make a person cry like this every day sit back and watch, and not at least try to help, it was as if it was what they wanted, finally what started as a wonderful exiting adventure turned to a nightmare, I looked at myself crying in the ladies room countless days, and asked myself, if it was worth all this, my god was everyday no matter where I went going to be like this,? And I always saw this beautiful woman looking back, tears running down her face the top of her dress soaked in tears, but she was so beautiful. I could not let her die, she was just starting to come to life, and I was going to continue to let her live. Thanksgiving and Christmas that year where the saddest ones of my life, holidays I once cherished I just wanted to go away. I felt I did not deserve anything and I wanted nothing, my wife was harsh and not sympathetic in anyway, just the same old better get a pay check, that's all I was good to her for, and I decided to file for unemployment, even though I quit, I felt I was forced to go, even though the company helped at first, They left me abandoned to hostile employees, And a boss who only saw it one way, his, So I asked for the papers to file and was told how surprised they where I would do that, and I said you know it should not have ended like it did something is just wrong here, I want a fair hearing, I never got one there, and I had an attorney who at the time was not involved fully but they were made aware of it, So I applied and at first was denied, it said I voluntarily quit, and had to appeal, so I did, and soon I was in a big office building in Boston waiting in a room when I look up and here comes the woman from personal with the companies head law consultant and my old boss, when I see them I can't hold the back tears. As hard as it was and as bad as the end was, Some of them I had known for years and felt befriended and I really lost part of my life there almost six of them, you start to feel like part of a family, And then you do something they don't like and make you leave, and in a way that lets you know they do not love you anymore, And now we are at the end of tables to argue over me getting a paycheck, we are allowed two hours I get the first then they get the last, then the board hears the report and makes a decision. We start! He asks me about my job who I am and why I am there. And before I know it in between the tears and questions I am asked and his head shaking in surprise, the two hours are up all going to me, He said I never in my life ever heard anything like this before! Ever! and slammed his book down shut, He then said we must return so you the employer can tell their side of this, but they did not come back, they had decided to stop and allow my unemployment payments, and after meeting with my attorney, we made an out of court settlement, small, but my lawyer said, I never ever saw a company abuse someone and discriminate someone so out right as horrible and as obvious as I have seen here, and I tell you honestly the length of time this went on 90 percent is expired you cannot do anything about it because you took too long to complain, but on the other hand I have enough to take them into court and teach them a lesson they will never forget, But let me tell you, it will take years it will be hard on you, you will get up there and be ripped to pieces by them again and for what? More money! but really not a lot more to make it worth it for what you will be put through, she said move on, let it go, I think you are a beautiful woman, forget those people and just go on with your life, you will relive this nightmare you just went through another ten years if they keep appealing, And from what I have seen, you are far too sensitive to handle it, I will do it! if you want, but let me warn you, it is going to be a long hard drawn out fight, and I will win, but it's you I worry about, you are way too sensitive, you need to grow a thicker skin, I said you are right I just want to move ahead and thanked her for all her good advice and her encouragement to move on, and that's what I did, I found a course to take in school, A medical assistant course, what I thought was a lot like being a nurse but was wrong, I wished later that I took the nurses course, but even so it was moving on and something new, and a woman's line of work, I pass my test to get approved for the college course and approved for the student loan, only one thing I needed now, I had to bring in a real copy of my high school diploma, and oh no guess what? It had my old name on it, so I say to myself this is the city, who will care? They must see this all the time. so I bring it in and all my name change documents to prove that's me on the diploma, the administrator is surprised and I get to joke a little, I say so I fooled you huh? she says yeah you did, I never would have known, I say thanks your nice to say that, I hope I really do look that good, and she says you look fine, you really do, and soon have a start date, but before I start my first day there, I get a call to go to the dean's office, a woman's is there with a couple others, she said, I just want you to know before you start and before you get settled in and can't get your money back, that this is what you want to do, I say I am sure I want to try at it, and she says that you are with a lot of tough city girls in here, this is not the suburbs, these girls will eat you up and spit you right out, they are street smart and most likely you won't fool many of them, you still want to try? I say yes, and then she says when it comes to your extern ship because we know about your situation and where you are in your transition, we are obligated to tell our clients your situation or we could be in Trouble because we do a lot of woman's clinics. And there is a right to know act and a woman has a right to know if a male is in the room especially alone, and although you have gotten as far as you have we still need to be aware of where we send you so no one gets offended just in case something goes wrong, So I say ok, and I start, and that's where there is a mistake them asking me my personal business and me being too honest and telling them, I did not have to tell them I was pre-op, I had a right to my own privacy and they invaded it and I was alone out there with no guidance and I did not know what to say, and there is always that reply if I lie, where are your surgical papers for proof, why, would I need those? And the school what a course! I never did lectures and wrote notes and had to keep up and do tests at the end each day and I really understood now why doctors write so lousy, I am so busy trying to learn I never even notice if anyone knows who or what I am, these young girls probably wonder what's with all the thick makeup at school, I had to use a cosmetic type called derma blend, people who have scars all over them or skin problems use it, actors because it lasts so long, And it hides that 5:00 shadow real well all day long, and it's very expensive, and hard to find, about seventy five dollars a month just for the foundation and sealer finishing powder, I still had electrolysis work to do and it is expensive and slow and to really get it to work you have to grow your beard out, So I had to time everything I did or I was busted, I flunk my first module, F a big one, F for school and F for me, I was so hurt I did not know I sucked that bad, and almost just gave up, and I just cried at my desk, it felt like I made the wrong choice and was now stuck with the bill, 4,000 dollars for nothing, but the teacher sees me in tears and says hang in don't give up, you are not the only one to fail half of the class failed, keep trying I will help you, and she gives me a big hug and says I also know about what you are going through, and I know that makes it harder for you, I said, how? she said they told me, I am your homeroom teacher, and will help you with anything you need, don't worry you will be fine you look just like the rest of them, blend in, don't stand out keep doing that, you'll make it. And I did I took all her advice and graduated with high honors. And what was so funny is I picked up a couple of the girls in the morning so they got to school on time, Ones I became friends with, I drove in and saved them waiting for the trains, and buses, In the morning getting ready for school they undressed and dressed right in front of me bare ass naked, just like I was one of the girls, what a good sign I passed well, That was a surprise and keeping a straight face the first few times that happened, is something I had to think about, I guess if I got by these tough city girls I would do ok, And I graduated way ahead in my class top ten in it what a nice feeling to succeed, finally my very first accomplishment for this little woman to be. But my extern ship was proven to be not at all what I hoped it would be, it was at a hospital in Boston, in the free clinic, all the homeless and poor people off the streets of Boston, and at first nothing to do. The first week I file papers but that's it, no clinical work, I do so much, so fast I run out of work, so I am on the floor all I do is stand there waiting, and waiting, all week and nothing, not even a blood pressure or a pulse check, temps nothing, they leave me standing there, 2'nd week the same, and I am starting to be concerned, I am supposed to be in training, doing something clinical, hands on, and all I do is stand here, so I confront the nurse, she said call your school. So I call and tell them, all they say is, this is all we could get you, just sit tight, it will soon be over and you will graduate, But I want to learn and get that hands on experience I like getting, well this is the best we can do for you, you're lucky we found you anything, I said you told them? They say yes, I say well they are holding me back, this is not fair, and they say just hang in there. So I go to the nurse and I tell her how it's upsetting to me that I just stand here all day doing nothing, She just looks at me, I look back, I say, I know you know, know what? She said, I said about me, the school told me they told you. Oh yes they did, if I was you I would get them in a lot of trouble for that because they had no right to. That's discrimination, they lied, we do not have to know your business, you represent yourself as a woman and you are legally one and I am sure everything you are doing everything is done legally I don't hold it against you at all, my hands are tied, she said by the way what makeup do you use it's fantastic, I say derma blend, she says no way, my sister uses that, and for the first time we talk. And she promised me Wednesday's she will have work for me. Wednesday is the day all the poor and homeless come in to have their leg ulcers cleaned and rewrapped, it has to be done right, she trains me, it's disgusting, and very smelly from the flesh that rots away from people under nourished or diabetic, where there varicose veins on their legs bundle up, and gets infected, turns into a large opening that will close if treated right, And it's medical work, and I do it, and soon this part of it is over. I don't go to my graduation as I am very upset and I wanted to wear the white robe the girls wore so bad, I had to wear the red one in high school the boys wore, and it meant a lot to me to be there just for that, and disappointed with the way they handled this whole extern ship I stayed home, but I get my diploma in the mail and start to look for work in the medical field, and one more thing I need to find another gender therapist, I let mine go, I felt at the end he could have and should have done more, the lines of communications where open, I signed release forms for him and the company doctor, should a problem arise and one did, and I asked for help, a simple phone call! at least an attempt, To try and solve that issue or any issue I had at the time as little or big as it may have been, instead of me suffering at the hands of what I now call a little monster of a boss, but all I got was they have to call me first, and they say he has to call us first, back and forth back and forth, I paid a lot of money he did not accept insurance, cash only, any document I needed to have typed up cost me money, not less than $150.00 that I would need for getting my name change and female on license, and I was with him almost 5 years maybe 6, and saw him about 20 times a year at one point, year at $100, a visit which went up to $120,00 to $140.00 if he had to move and pay higher rent he never had a stable office and moved a lot, and the one time I need him the most He is not there, the one real crucial time I need a helping hand from him, He deserts me, I don't know why. Maybe his credentials are not what he claims, he said if I got surgery I would be the first he ever had from start to finish, and I was so close, I arranged for surgery march 22 the spring of that following year, I had the money I was in touch with a surgeon. I just need to get a few documents and pay the money and fly out to the hospital. It was in the U.S I cannot at this time 20 years later tell where or who was the hospital and dr. But it all just fell apart I suffered a long emotional breakdown afterwards, This journey, it's hard dangerous, and scary to be out there all alone, and I was told I had to have a job and prove I was still emotionally stable enough for the surgeon and all of his psychological staff to clear me, and I was an emotional wreck. I was not ready, this sudden stop and turn around in my life was so much a strain on my heart from it being so broken into pieces from all of this, I needed to recover just so I could think about what just happened, one day I am a successful man working in a Tool And Die shop taking care of a family next thing I am a transgendered person all alone out there all by myself, wondering where I was going to go next, and just touch my feet back on the ground, to make sure all of this was not just a bad dream, And I was unemployed and that was another requirement, I understand they want you to have a job, but all the hell I just went through was a shock, It took six months to get a real hold of myself again, I barely remember those first six months after, I have no idea how I made it through school like I did, it was like a dream, I could not believe it was over, all those years there and overnight I am sitting in a desk at school, and I know barely one person if any missed me the day after I left that factory, I still had my doctor for the hormone therapy but I was out there on my own, and soon he died, He had a heart attack right at his desk, His son took his place but soon he moved away, I had to start all over again and find another medical doctor and gender therapist first, And get back into a reassignment program with someone else, you can buy hormones on the street and find shady doctors and go it alone, but not me I want to do it right, be a legal female, and have very prominent educated doctors to support me that really care, lucky I had enough hormones to get buy another 9 months, vand when I ran out my primary care doctor wrote me one with a few refills, but said he will only this one time, he said he wants me with someone who knows what they are doing, and he is so right, I am really glad that he made me go back out and do it right, and I find one, in Brookline near my school and a nice "woman", and this time she finds me a medical doctor closer to home, the others where way out in the northern part of the state, about an hour ride this is, 25-30 minutes, and his approach to hormones is, different he gives me a male hormone block, It's safer, less chance of a stroke, plus the female hormones at half the dose, and it is quite an improvement my breast grow another cup size in months I feel the pressure in them like they want to burst, I love it, I love any feeling that is a feeling I am changing, and I lose a lot more body hair everywhere, I shave my legs once a month, except that damn beard, though it slowed it down and it's not so rough anymore, A lot of it is gone, from electrolysis, the change is great for me. Even my face is changing, my cheeks are getting puffier and they are high any way this really makes them show up nice, and my erections are going away, not even when I wake in the morning, and it so good to get that to stop, along with the urge to go out to the kitchen draw and get out a sharp knife, and I get a new job! One I am so excited about. I am going to work for the American Red Cross, I was so proud of myself, I felt like a proud little girl scout, I am always so happy when I really get to do a woman's "thing" I was always left out and had to watch what I wanted to come and do, those feelings are like a good trumpet player who watches a parade and a band goes by and he has his trumpet in his hand as he watches them and he wants to go and join in and play along, I never in a million years thought I would work for them and here I was hired and in training to go to blood donation sites and place the needle in people willing to give blood, to help others in need, what a change and a big step up from what I was doing before, always to me a step up I never took off any crowns stepping down from a man, instead I grew beautiful wings to fly, And also another important thing! a grandparent, my oldest daughter had a son with her boyfriend, and I still say boy, this was no man at all, And also we had found a house to buy, not one I wanted, it needed to much work, But my wife and daughter found it and they really wanted it, I was just happy to move and get out of that project we were in, my daughter and my wife really believed this guy would help, not me! I knew he would not, I heard him with my daughter up in her room as he was beating her one night, telling her go ahead and get this new home, you and your parents won't see one nickel of mine ever, I will never help you with the baby! Ever! you are on your own, you are just a nasty little white whore, that's all you will ever be, and I heard the beating and called the police, she denies everything, she said he never touched her, after the police left saying there was nothing they could do and I don't know why she was 17, I told them what I heard, But they say I had to have seen it, I was walking upstairs disgusted with her for that, and she punches me in the back of the head. And says don't you ever call police on us again mind your own business, I threw her out, him too, and the police where right outside, I said get out or I get him back here, but later my wife lets them back in as usual, telling me we need them to help with the house, we are buying, I could snap and go crazy, It's good I just sold all my guns, my kids where older and looking through closets, even though I took every precaution in the book it was not enough, guns don't belong around children, I believe we should be able to all own one but with children in the house the safety and security of the weapon is more than crucial it is a moment gone wrong that will destroy an entire family and even a community, he is thankful mine are gone, what will it take to get her and my dumb daughter to believe he does not care at all, He is just using us, I can't get rid of him myself, they will bring him back and give him a tummy rub, I believed putting a restraining order on him myself would have made me the one who had to leave, and if I did my two younger babies would get neglected and abused, and I am so glad I stayed, the temptations to just flee at that time in my life were so strong, but I really felt the danger around my two youngest children, and later in life in their twenties they finally tell me that one of the things my oldest daughter and her bad girl friend would do to them if they didn't like dinner or lunch, was hold their head over the kitty litter box and shoved their faces in if they struggled or refused to eat, what was she thinking. and that friend of hers was awful, the whole family was, and my daughter was always with them, they bribed her with food and amusement parks so there daughter had a friend, no one else in the neighborhood would go near her, and this is one of the things brought into my home from outside, I could not believe some of the abuse they told me about. and as intimate as I want to be in my book about myself I can't say everything when it comes to my children like that, and other things they told me I will not even want to remember, thank god for giving me the strength to hang in there for them, how painful it was to stay And to take them with me and start out like this was going to be too hard for them, and a possible custody battle, so I went to work to get away from them all, and I loved the red cross what I liked best is the dress code, non-casual, dresses whenever possible is one thing they tell us and that's fine with me, we move into the new house I am unpacking and about to have the worst weekend of my life, it's may, memorial day weekend and it's Friday, the truck is unloaded and I am going through the boxes to unpack, when my oldest daughter comes in and tells me I need the camera for the baby, he looks so cute, right now I need to get a picture quick, and I say you have to give me a few minutes. I don't know where the camera is at the moment I will have to look for it, look at all the boxes, no she says! Now! You get f;ing camera right now! And I say no I will look in a minute, she says now! I said get that f'ing camera now, I said no! Now I will not even look for it, get out, leave the house, I am busy, she said no! I will not get out and you will get that f'ing camera now. And she came in through the door swinging punches at me, I am on the floor, going through a box, I am trying to stand and block off her punches at the same time, it's hard she is swinging wildly at me and she knows how to throw a punch, I taught her how, and she took Aikido lessons with her sisters, I just get to my feet and she knows now she has had it, I am up! And ready. she stops and turns and runs up the stairs, I just go back to unpacking I know of nothing being wrong, But I hear her yelling to someone that I beat her up, and then about five minutes later I hear sirens and then police coming in the house they say did you just get in a fight with someone, I said no, they say who hit the girl I say what girl? They say are you her dad? I say yes, they say what just happened, tell them all I know is I was unpacking my daughter wanted a camera and I couldn't find it fast enough for her, she got upset I told her to get out of the house she said no and she started to try and hit me, I just blocked her punches, what's your name, I said Cynthia, they say Cynthia? You're her dad, I say yes! I changed my name, I am undergoing a sex change, oh really, they all just stare at me then say turn around, I am cuffed brought down and booked for assault, on the way out I see an ambulance, I am surprised I say what happened? They say you know, you just beat your daughter up real bad and I said what? I said I did not I said she attacked me all I did was block some punches, They said shut up we heard enough, and we have heard all we need to know, we are arresting you, They never even read me my rights, until after I was already locked up, and reminded them, they kept me for three days locked in a cell over the long weekend, I refused to eat and drink and they did not care, every day three times a day they slid burger king meals under the little slot under the door and I just kicked it back out, but the smell of it did not make me hungry but made me think of my two younger babies at home, we always went to burger king, we liked it better than McDonalds, I cried every time they brought it, I got no help or support from anyone I had one lawyer who said if my wife signed an agreement to put a lien on our home for 5000, he would help get me right out, but she would not do it, the police brought people in and showed me off like I was some kind of animal, they would bang on my door and open a little slot and say look it's a Mr. Cynthia we got in here, Hi Mr. Cynthia and walk away laughing, kicking my door to aggravate me, I wanted to die in there, and if I did, not one person in that police station would have noticed till they did a bed check, every 8 hours, or came to harass me, I only wondered only about my two youngest daughters at home who I knew where being frightened and bullied now by their older sister and boyfriend Now boasting over there achievement, and that in the back of my oldest daughter and perhaps even my wife's minds they may have hoped that I would give this up, And think it was not worth it, and blame myself for being the one bringing all the violence and pain and confusion into our home, I knew my two babies at home where scared and alone in a new home away from their friends and neighbors, that just a few days ago they were out in the play areas playing with, And that gave me strength to live. If not for them I would have let myself die in that cell that weekend, I am sure, and not one person I know or who was there would have cared, I ate no food and had no water except when I took medicine for angina and seizures. My wife was no help at all, she could have told the police my daughter was a very abusive child and was lying and she herself had been abused and beaten by her and got me out earlier, helped somehow just helped, even with that lawyer, but she did nothing, no one was there. I had no idea what even happened, but later find out that when my daughter ran up the stairs the pitch in the roof was low at the top of the landing and she banged her head running up them and got a real bad scrape then called the police and said I did it! And because I was a transgendered person I was arrested, I was guilty till proven innocent, what a disgrace the police dept. is in the town I moved to and now live, and I am not ashamed or afraid to say that in my book, I was arrested for who I was, not for what really happened, no one stuck up for me at all, not even my wife who had gotten 38 stitches in her mouth from this girl, no one, abandoned again, in the court house jail I was first confined alone I looked like a woman. I had breasts and woman clothes on, they refused to even let me clean up before court, Then the jailer throws a guy into my cell and he gets upset And says hey let me out! There's a woman in this cell you made a mistake!

The jailer says that's not a lady, the guy stares at me, I say hi what you in for? and he walks over and sits down and says wow you really a dude, I say yes I am, he said I think that's interesting I never met anyone like you before, I heard of it, but never met anyone, and he talked to me a half hour very polite and very interested in what I was doing, I told him anything he asked we became friends, I told him why I was here, he felt bad for me like he really understood. So it was not too bad, at least that part, though I do believe if I ever got a lawyer and the civil liberty union after some of these rights violations I had happen to me,

There would have been a lot of regrets to some people, but I wanted to still protect those two small babies I had at home I thought more of them and their pain more than any of mine and the publicity that would envelope the solitude and quiet private life I so wanted, and never in my life will I ever forget or forgive them for this, ever, and I had to call out sick for the red cross, a long week end out was unheard of, this was not good, I was in trouble, I was a newer employee too, when I got in and told my lead person what happened and she knew what a problem my daughter has been her heart went out for me, I was crying my heart out, they just sent me back home, They at this time had no idea I was in a gender reassignment program or anything yet but they would find out and how they do and what happens because of it is horrible, but by now at home the DSS has caught up to my daughter and some justice is served to me, they are not done with my daughter yet, she is given an ultimatum lose the boyfriend get a restraining order or we take your baby, they give her one week to make her decision and tell her what day and time they will return to get there answer, or the take her baby, I just arrive from work and she is outside with the baby in her arms and they come, the Police and the DSS and a plains clothes detective laughs and points at me in my dress and says That's the "dad" no wonder, and laughs. I look at him and get him to look at my hand just by wiggling it around a little bit, and I give him the finger, real quick, I have had enough from these guys, he wasn't too happy, so what, and then they ask her well what did you decide restraining order or we take your baby, She says no! no restraining order, I won't get one because you are making me, if you weren't trying to make me do it I would on my own, and they say, look right now we will still give you that opportunity to get that order we don't want to take your baby we are here to help you, tell us what you will do, him or the baby, we don't believe you will go get one on your own, you would have by now, Guess what she does, she hands over her baby, right in front of me, She refuses to comply with the DSS they fear for the baby and the mothers safety, more the baby, and she chose that nasty, woman beating, low life boyfriend. Over her own child, Who is sitting upstairs watching television, waiting for the decision my daughter was to make, him or the baby, and I can't believe what I am seeing and hearing with my own ears and eyes right in front of me. I lost so much respect for her that day, And will never take it back, there is no excuse, and I will never forgive her for doing that, what a foolish child everyone was there to help, and even after that, her baby gone, the violence continues, till finally they are fighting with tire irons on the street smashing each other's car windows out, swinging them wildly at each other, and a neighbor calls the police and later he will be a witness in court to seal his doom, they are both arrested, it is the last time she lives with us, we threw her out, there's no baby now, to blackmail me with, and I walk over to my neighbor. and I apologize for my daughter and her boyfriend and I thank him, I tell him he has just saved my daughter's life. And I hope someday she will grow up and someday herself come to you and thank you herself for what you did, he told me he was so frightened for his own children also, that they could have gotten hurt from the incident, that's how far they took it, And the strangest of all things, the Jailer at the court house The DA, that wanted to prosecute me and try to make my daughter look like such a victim and it was me, I was the victim, he even used the press against me, he said I will tell your entire life to the press you won't have a private moment for years, I will put you all over the news, and another jailer who pushed me up the stairs and whacked me with his club while I was cuffed and shackled and weak from not eating and drinking all died within a few years of that time I was there two had heart attacks and one was murdered, Hoping that part of my life with my daughter is over but it's not, The Red Cross is going great till one day all my fingers tips are swollen I squeezed one and puss popped out along the edges of my nails, I had just switched to a powdered glove, we ran out of non-powdered and it was a reaction, I went back to the non-powdered. Two weeks later when we finally got some, but the infection kept getting worse. All my nails got soft and cracked and my fingertips also, An hour or two with gloves on and my hands where burning, cracked, itching and bleeding, I had lost all my fingernails they just peeled away, I showed my supervisor and reported it, I was wearing bandages on each fingertip, the doctor looks at my hands, I tell him what I do for work and the first thing right away he says, you can't sue, I said what? Did you say sue? He said yes, you can't sue, whatever do you mean? and why would you say that?, I just want to get better and go back to work, ok he said then I will run tests, he took samples and the results he claims are psoriasis and not glove related, and two other doctors say the same thing, first thing they say when you tell them what you do for work is, you can't sue, I never in my life had three doctors in a row say that first thing right out of their mouth, it's as if they don't want to admit there is a problem out there, why all of a sudden are other people having trouble. And why all of sudden are they trying new types of rubber and plastics? and trying new powders, after taking some time away they heal and when I go back and put gloves back on within days it's returning, and I lost my sense of touch, it's as if my fingers where burnt I lost the feeling at the tips and my skills and amount of blood I was supposed to collect each month fell behind, finding a vein that was not visible was getting more difficult, touch and feel was so important, and I was losing mine. My first ever review was bad, and it hurt, this was job I really wanted, I made lots of friends, the shifts where crazy but I traveled all over the state, and I could wear anything nice, and dresses where my choice, Then We did a union place in S.Boston, and I got a funny reception when I returned there a second time, seemed that I was looked at more closely by the hostess but I ignored it, it's just me being paranoid. A week later a woman comes to me at another drive and looks right at me and she says, I know what you are going through, I was shocked, I just stared back at her in shock and she knew she scared me, and at break she came over to me and said I am so sorry if I scared you, I know I did, that was wrong of me, Relax I am a gay woman I have seen and I know people like you, I admit you had me fooled a long time and it's not your looks that gave you away, you actually look very good, it's actually something that I heard there is a real strange rumor going around and I really need to tell you because they are openly discussing it at blood drives, Do you remember when we went to the real big blood drive in S. Boston? In the union building, they say you used the men's room, and you stood and peed in the urinal along with the men, in a dress! I was so shocked, I said no way! I never did that, she said that's the rumor, I am not kidding you, I did not know what to think, the only one there I used was a handy cap bath room, and I always sit, doesn't matter, most of my life I have anyway, Only at school as a child if I really had to, but peeing in front of people ever since a small child is about impossible, I have some disorder with that, I don't' know what, but it never went away, I still have it, sitting is the only way I can really pee, not that it bothers me at all, I talk to the woman who trained me soon as I can, she is a black woman, One of their first to work for them, she has been there a long time, and we became very close, I went to her and I said let me ask you, have you heard any unusual rumors about me, and she grinned and said yes, yes I have, and she repeated the same story, I was just horrified, I said no, no way, I admitted I was in a sex change program and was pre-op but I told her I never used the men's room, and that I don't know how this came out, this is very viscous, she said what bathroom did you use there and I said the handicap down stairs, she huh, huh, Well we have had trouble with the men there peeping through holes in the ladies room, they must have one there also. I said if they do it's in a real good spot, I am so careful, which means someone is looking up every woman's privates real good and up close, I said I really need to tell someone this, she said look, I am a black woman and very old I got 20 years on you, I know discrimination and how horrible it is, the people in management here are the most prejudice people ever, If you go in with this you are going to open up a can of worms, and not just with the red cross but this is South Boston and these union members, some are people you don't want to mess with, leave it, I will help where I can, but a lot of damage is done, and she said I honestly feel for you I know how much you love this job, but I believe your days maybe numbered now, and she was right soon my performance was under the microscope, I was watched everywhere I went, when I went to get my hands looked at again they even tried to sneak in a drug test, one I would have done but I arrived late, and did not even know about it, But I realized they were looking for a way to get rid of me, what did a drug test have to do with my hands, Also at a drive in Quincy a woman comes in, talks to a nurse there, they know each other, they are friends, and the woman is a woman from my daughters old color guard and she did not like me or my daughter, My daughter got the spots her daughter wanted, so there was a lot of rivalry, she came in to I.D me, put me right there, after that it was about over and that along with some damn peeping tom, a damn perverted little bastard had destroyed my job and career, It was horrible. I loved this job I cried for months after I lost this one, it was hard leaving a job you traveled to so many places a lot, you remember a collage of pictures and memories that overwhelm you, for months, not like remembering the office chair you sat at, Some girls and woman finding out I was who I was really embraced me and took me right in and accepted me and I got the most sincere hugs you could ever ask for, and they did their best to help, but there numbers not big enough, I miss them, awful bad, the last few months I saw them and got a hug goodbye from the ones who knew and cared and loved this person

I shared with them, I will always miss them so much, It was clear in the upper ranks they did not want me, and the next flair up with my hands was so bad they put me on disability, and said they will bring me back when I heal real well or they may have to just keep me on a different job. But I knew they were getting rid of me for good, I tried a typing test and missed by one letter each time on the time it took and I had so much trouble with my fingers trying, but that was not good enough, I thought these people who worked for such an organization had compassion, but what I really found out was the donor part of the red cross is there money maker and if you are in any way interfering or disrupting a blood drive and not keeping up, out you go, I had a good reason to sue them, but it was the red cross I could not bring myself to sue an organization I felt was there to help people, I was shocked to hear a few years later. The higher people in management that gave me a hard time and threw me out so coldly, had been indicted for fraud and stealing money, and were found guilty, now I wish I had sued them, I was on disability and I got a part time job pumping gas, not very lady like, But I need the money for the mortgage and all my bills, And I did that almost a year and left when it was just too cold out and the pay was ok but the station I worked at made you wash every windshield of a customer's car, and you had to, he had spies come and check on you, and he got a lot of business, I was working like crazy there, and it was getting too cold for me, I found a job at a super market it started out good but the holidays where coming when you spend 8 hours sliding turkeys down the counter and bag them all day, that's hard work, and we never had any one to bag, all the baggers, they went out to get carriages but what they were really doing was hiding behind cars drinking beer and smoking pot, I had just a met a new therapist at my depression clinic, the medical doctor was always so busy and she wanted me with someone I could at least spend 30-45 minutes with, a session, and she says I think I have found someone for you, the medical doctor and owner of the clinic was a real sweetheart, very small and petite as they come but also a full-fledged colonel in the army, A real tough little lady, she to me was an inspiration as a woman, if I was born the correct gender in the beginning I would have wanted a mentor like her, I have known her since she started her new practice I meet my new therapist, my gender therapist is far away and I only see her a few times a year, mostly because of my hours that I work, And I meet Ingrid a nice kind friendly little German woman. with a strong accent and a real pleasant smile and we talk briefly our first session, and she says right away that she has no experience with gender identity issues, and at first is surprised when I tell her I am a transsexual, she was not told, and I get pass her eye test, she had one patient she treated for anxiety but it was the reversal of what I was, it was a woman becoming a man, and that was all she had and she felt she would not be a lot of help to me, I said is anyone here experienced with someone like me? And she said no I don't think so, I said how do you feel about learning what it's like for me and what I go through along with all the other problems life hands out to me,? Smiling I said after all there is the human factor also, I am one of those too, and I do have anxiety and panic attacks and depression, and no one around to talk to or share my thoughts with, if you are willing to learn and follow me along as I go I would be happy to see you, and so we agreed to meet, I wake up later one morning and my left arm is asleep, all numb I can barely move it, I try working at the grocery store, and it's very difficult, just trying to hold dollar bills and count them is almost impossible and a lot of work, I thought to myself I must have pinched a nerve, and then I stutter a little, but I have to keep working, I have an appointment with a Neurologist about my back, and neuropathy's I have, and migraines, And I have just had an x-ray of my brain looking for reasons for headaches, so I just wait, months go buy and my arm just kind of hangs there, but I keep using it and it gets just a little better, but not too good, Then one night on my way home I stop to get gas, a little man comes to the window, very polite, and grinning away, says your cute, anyone tell you, you are a beautiful woman, I just say no, not often, and smile back, he keeps smiling and says how much, I say give me ten dollars he said ok, he puts the nozzle in my car and comes back making small talk again, he touches my shoulder, I just look at him he says again your cute and bends down and real quick kisses me on the cheek, I was surprised, this has never happened, I start to get a little wary, and the pump stops, that loud pop when they stop. He looks at it then looks at me and again says I think you are very, very beautiful, and now I am getting anxious, I look in my side mirror again, the pump is still in my car, I feel like I want to flee suddenly, I get so paranoid all my warning flags are up, but I can't, if I do I will rip the hose out of the car, and I haven't paid yet, so I give him his money, he puts it in with the rest of his money and he is so slow, just looking at me while he does this, then he reaches in my car quickly puts his hand on my stomach and slides his hand up and squeeze's my left breast I was stunned completely, nothing like this has ever happened to me before, I had to get out of this one fast, I knew I could just get out of my car and beat his ass but then if he ran to the nozzle and sprayed gas on me and threw a match, I would get burnt to death, If I flee he will say I took off without paying, I had to think real quick and a lot of thoughts raced through my mind this is new! I am learning things so unexpectedly out here, my left arm was still weak and he could have a knife or anything on him, but he said, ok? You ok? I say yeah ok, I got to go, he said you married? I said yes!! I am going to see my husband now! He says ok, bye, and goes over and removes the nozzle and I drive off, still in a daze, what had just happened? Did I just get molested? By some creep! Is this part of being a woman? Wow, what a horrible thing that is to have happen, I felt very awkward, and a little pissed off, part of me wanted to go back and kick his ass, I don't say anything to anyone and I keep thinking about it, and I think, if he has done it to me is he doing it to other woman? Should this guy get reported? I am really unsure what happened and what to do, but lucky for me I see Ingrid soon and in the next couple days, I tell her what just happened, she said yes you got molested, unfortunately it's part of what we woman deal with, but we don't have too. This guy needs to be stopped, I ask if I should see the police and she says yes right away, he may be doing this to other woman, help stop him, I go to the police, the next day, I ask to speak to a woman detective, and she says what's up? I tell her, and she asks is it the gas station near the old shoe store? a little guy with a moustache?, I said yes, she said we know about him, and you're not the first this week to come in, she asks my name and says I remember you, she said you're the one who had a sex change or something right?

And I say yes, how do you know all this? Do you remember me from somewhere? She said I am the one who spoke to at your home from the hospital incident. When your daughter kicked you then you threw her out and she went and said you beat her up, that's you? I say yes, she said you look great, how is your daughter still? I say worse, she says too bad, sometimes we need to let people in our lives go, I hope all this is working out for you, it takes a lot of courage to do what you are doing, I really appreciate you coming in, we want this guy and with you now we can go and get him, now we have another witness with the same story, I tell her he is very cunning he traps you there, she said how, how did you feel trapped, I said he leaves his pump in your tank you cannot drive off without ripping it out, and she said oh! ok, yes that's not to good, I understand why anyone would be afraid, After that I never saw him again I don't know where he went but it's good to know he is off the street, and I did something to make it safer for woman to get there gas, as time goes along it's pretty quiet my daughter is gone from the house, Her boyfriend gets a five year term, and after seven months is allowed to have her baby back, But she does not come back home, she got an apartment with the help from the state, and puts her baby in a day care, I go into my job at the super market and a woman boss said are you quitting? I said no, she said I heard you where, I said no, then a girl I had told a few weeks ago I was not feeling well my arm was weak and I was very dizzy and tired, my back ached terribly and I just said I don't think I can make it too much longer, just out of the blue, I didn't even remember saying it, had just approached and said yes you did! You said you want to quit. And that's why you're missing work, I said no I just really don't feel well, and the lady said I believe her! leave, give me your uniform and leave, you just quit, I was shocked, I couldn't believe this, another job gone from a rumor, and a silly one at that, some kids word against mine, there was more to it than that, One of this girls friends would say here comes tootsie every time she saw me, and now I knew why, I got read, And it was hard to pass, as a woman in that horrible uniform I had to wear and the lighting, it was so bright in there, I was lucky I passed at all, I had only but about 2-3 years out there and kids are hard especially girls who look for every flaw of your character, and I worked with two who just did not want me around I guess, so I went home, But I had one experience at the supermarket that I will never forget, it was a man who worked there in stock, one day he came in with a handful of flowers and handed them to me and grabbed me and gave me a big kiss, right on the lips, then told me he was so in love with me, and that he had to have me, would I please go out soon on a date? I was stunned, I never had that happen, either, all these new adventures, I just thanked him, I said you are so sweet but I am married and he was so sad, I think about it and I always wondered how my reaction to an event like that would be when it happened if ever, and I enjoyed it, I felt very womanly and it was so cute, I will always remember that, My favorite part of being a woman is my memories way of remembering moments like that, falling in love myself or another, I remember my first time ever by sight, and as soon as I saw her, it was at a funeral, she came in with another man, I was single, and I thought who she was with was her husband, she came over and spoke to me as I sat, it was my Fathers, Fathers funeral, she had the softest voice I ever heard she spoke in a whisper and her large round eyes drew you in, every move she made was delicate as her soft whispering voice, I fell in love in an instant I never believed it possible, I found she was a distant relative second cousin to my Fathers cousin, she looked a lot like one of us, later at another funeral I would see the man she came with, and he was alone, I asked my mother who this man was and she said the brother of the nice woman he was always with second cousin of your father that just died, she was so sensitive and fragile, that when she had to go in for a routine operation got herself so upset she had a heart attack and died, I wish I had known the first time I met her, it was her brother she was with, he never left her side, she was just too delicate, she was on the very high side of the female spectrum, to fragile and easily broken, much like myself only I have come trapped inside the body of a man, and I do not fit in here but it may be why I lived as long as I did, and that is what I love so about my woman's heart the emotions all cluttered inside that on some days when I need them they flutter throughout my mind in a swarm of butterflies, anyway I was denied unemployment, they said I quit. And I never did, and not worth the 26 dollars a week to fight it, I finally see my neurologist, the x-rays, are there and when I return I got a surprise, I had had a stroke, it scared me so bad to hear him say that, a stroke,? That's bad, have you ever gotten told of a condition like that, one that almost killed you? It's terrifying to hear a doctor say that, it is similar to how you feel when you realize your gender is crossed over, and it will repeat itself if you fight it or deny yourself the truth, and soon a long list of health problems where to follow. Earlier before buying the house, we had a lot of snow the year before, I was shoveling constantly and one day I came in felt a horrible pain in my chest. It put me right on the floor, I said I think I'm having a heart attack, my wife looks at me and says your fine get off the floor there's nothing wrong with you.

And I say yes there is! I never had a pain like this it felt like I was slowly being crushed. Like an elephant was slowly pushing his big wide foot down on me. I relax and after a few moments it's gone but they keep returning, not as heavy but very noticeable. I tell my cardiologist, who brushes it off, he was treating me for Mitro valve prolapse and was acting very casual, oh you again, how many times do I have to tell you, you are ok, and I say this really hurt! it put me on the floor, So he says let's do a stress test right here in the office, I get hooked up and start up, ok at first, I can barely hang on, he is so surprised, he was just leaning against the wall expecting a routine test and then this, an emergency, he runs over looks at the scope I am hooked up to and says quick put this under your tongue and a nurse runs to help hold me up. He says my god! that's your heart, he is so surprised, I had complained so much but he never caught it, now he had, and he couldn't believe his own eyes, he did a cardiac cathedra later, He went through the artery in my leg and ran a scope up into my heart and said if I say cough, you better cough, ok, I look up at the screen I see my heart and all the vessels as I watch the probe make its journey, All of a sudden I get hot all over like someone just dropped an electric blanket on me, on super-hot, and I here cough, cough, quick cough, and I freeze I get scared I can't cough, look over to my left and a nurse is running with defibrillator paddles and looking right at me. I got so scared when I saw her coming I coughed, real fast, and the heat went right down and I started cooling down again to that hospital room cool temp, he pulls out the cathedra and says I see what's wrong, you have very tiny arteries, they are not blocked just very tiny, and they spasm, we all have spasms in our vessels, and arteries, But yours being so tiny they close up and stop blood and oxygen from getting to your heart, they are so small that doing this procedure is too risky, I got stuck up there and for a minute did not think I could remove the cathedra, don't ever get another one you may not live through it, he prescribed a timed release nitro-stat to keep my arteries dilated, I had one adjustment in my dose to get it right but I would have a few overnights at the hospital till it was under control, all this was just too much, I have been getting hit with all these health problems and on top of it. I am going through a sex change, where do I find the strength and courage? it's inside me, the desire to become a woman and be who I am was not going to be stopped by anything, even death, even being so suicidal all the time, I hung on, with hope all the time a little bit of hope shining through somewhere kept me going, I was always so suicidal every day, I thought of this a lot like being a prisoner I see myself hanging by my neck or pulling the trigger to a gun at my head, planning and dreaming of a way to end this misery on this planet, but I also have a strong desire to grow, to become me, all these years of hurt and wondering why, why me? Of all the things to be thrown at you it had to be this. I never remember it ever being different. I just keep going, I just keep plugging along, I just go get a newspaper and I find a job, it's a few towns over and they need a tool and die maker + mechanic, ok, tool and die maker part is easy, except! I had sold most of my precise measuring tools, out of fear that sitting around they would rust and change from climate changes if not stored right for a long time, and not be what I would ever need to go back to do the work I have done, I would need all brand new ones of the best brands and quality to match up to the work I did, and that I never thought I would return to such a male dominated field again, but I was good at it, about 15 years of my life was invested into those skills. Why not try and see how this works out. I apply the interview goes well I am asked questions only a very experienced tool maker could answer, This guy is really surprised, at how much a woman knows, on that subject, he talked more than just shop he went right into engineering, and used words that he really pulled out of the hat so to speak, and new school I am more old school, he knew what to ask all around, and I knew it all, he said I need to check your references and then you need a physical and if that goes good we will see, I got a few guys I am looking at but to tell you the truth you seem to be the most experienced person I have talked to so far, it looks good, can you handle a shop? I say what do you mean? He says the guy's, you know? The language, I laughed at that one, Was he listening, (NO) where did he think I learned what I knew? It will be them blushen not me I said. I get hired, all he said was get a roll around tool box, Mostly I want you to have is mechanics tools, most of the work is repairing machines the die work is small and very repetitious, and we have tools here you can use, I had a lot of mechanic tools from all the auto work I did and still did. It's a large plant they make file folders mostly foreigners work there, the work is fast and heavy all day long, same thing over and over, when pay day came most of the men hid from their wives and girlfriends who came to get money for their children, and pay the rent, but they had gambling debts and they all ate well off the canteen trucks and ran up high tabs, but there children ate little, and worried they would have the lights on to watch television when they got home, what a disgrace, how men suck, I learned one thing and that is men treat woman terribly. Not all of them, there are a few good ones but most of them are real rats, And on this side I hear a lot of woman's complaints, they are so right to say a lot of the things they do, and how they feel, they are right to complain for themselves and their babies, it's a man's world, and I am about to learn that! Again! I have more skills than the man I will work with on the tool and die end of the company; he is not even a half descent machinist never mind a Tool and Die maker. But he is a man and because he is, The choices made actually take half the jobs away from the company by the time they lay me off, and it's all that male ego stuff, the dies they ran there, made the steel part of the file folder that when you put it in your draw it hangs, the press is a 500 ton hydraulic, it builds up its force at the last inch of its stroke as it hits bottom resistance it builds up tonnage and quickly to push through the steel, not like a manual that hits with shock, like a punch and snaps the parts through causing more out of shape or bowed conditions, and the components in the die are all made of carbide a very strong steel, it last's ten times longer than regular tool steels, but if hit wrong will crack like glass, you have to have a lot of experience with it or you will do a lot of expensive damage, and maybe injure or kill someone, and there is where I will struggle not with the die's but with the "men" in charge, of making the decisions about what to repair in a die, I make all the suggestions I want, But they fall on deaf ears, the company wanted to increase business by developing a system they could make these rods and coat the ends with a white plastic that is melted with micro wave heat, all this happens fast, They want 350 strokes a minute which gives the 1400 rods a minute the die is built to make four with each stroke, and two presses so they would get 2800 rods a minute, to run that fast the timing of the die has to be perfect, You can adjust everything else around the die to get what you want, but to actually get the parts out of the die and run that fast, the die has to be timed perfect, It's like a giant sewing machine only running steel through it instead of thread the basic timing in the dies at this factory are terrible, the first things you learn as a die maker are ignored, they play with and adjust everything they adjust readjust, separate rolls of steel, they even went out and spent 5,000 on a metal hardness tester made by Rockwell to check to see if it was the steel, they go over and over and over it, but they cannot get the dies to run off the parts, I tell what I can do to fix them, they say they have their best "man" on it, I say he has not done this right, but he said he did so that counts, no matter what, they or I do with the press and everything around it, A product would not run constantly, we had meeting after meeting after meeting, I stuck to what I believed was wrong with the dies and at the last meeting when it was decided if we would both get to work on the dies, I am voted out, no! only "he" will, he is the only one that will repair the dies, and the project fails, the president of the company says enough, we want everything back at the mother factory, this line is down and along with that about 50 percent of their work planned for the future, it all went out the door, the guy who did the die work quit soon after, but they still had a quota to fill and all the dies where down, so they tell me to fix them, and it's my job I would like to say go "F" yourself, My Boss says go ahead try to fix them I don't dare look. He walks over when I have a die apart three of the mechanics are with me, all the top three, and the boss comes and rattles off real technical instructions at me, and I say yes to everyone, and ask questions just as technical back, they look at me after "the boss" leaves and they say did you really understand everything he said? We have no idea what any of that even meant. I said I know every detail just watch me, and the highest one there next to my boss just looks at me and said, You really know your shit don't you? I said yes, and you are all about to see it, my boss that hired me, He came over when I was sitting the die in the press, and said I can't bear to look! Say your prayers I am out of here and left! He really thought I would fail and wanted me to fail. But I prove otherwise, Every roll of steel in the plant runs through the press in days not weeks or months like before "days", And without adjusting or playing with anything around the machine, once I put that die in and set up the press the operator stood there in amazement, as rods flew out and filled the conveyor belts, all the rejected rolls of steel that we were told would never run, ran, my boss was stunned and embarrassed, a "woman" just showed up a group of technical engineers and mechanics that struggled for six months to get what I took days to complete, I had the last word, A Woman can do a man's job, with my makeup, my red lipstick, blush, ponytail and polished nails I blew them all away, and they knew it, it was right there in front of them, and you can believe my boss got an ass chewing, but it was too late to save any jobs, The presses where on their way out and I was getting my pink slip soon, But I was not that disappointed I had scored a big win for woman, I felt this time

I left a winner, a big winner, But also a real big disappointment with management and how they handled my exit, when I started this job, again I had to get the family plan so I had to go in and explain my marriage as two woman, not yet legal in this state, I did not say pre or post-op I feel I don't have to, but I did find if you hold back they can ask for proof you had surgery, I don't know if that has changed, I hope so, upon cleaning out my locker and walking out after saying goodbye to everyone I was friends with, I heard the woman in personal, she was in the shop with all the guys I just worked with, and I heard her say, so! Did any of you know Cynthia used to be a man, very teasingly, I was so upset, I asked her not to, I knew some of the guys developed small crushes on me, they brought me in little gifts and helped with heavy things and helped me learn to fix machines, all with manners and respect, except that one guy who thought he was a Tool and Die Maker but he was not, he must have worked in laundry, And I warned her if she said anything she would cause hurt feelings maybe even anger and depression, I said it would or could have very bad consequences, but she did not listen, when I heard her go in and tell them I was so mad I thought about suing them for all the discrimination, I would have made a fortune, but it's not me, I don't want to leave a trail of lawsuits behind me everywhere I go, but I came back to visit when I was working again, all three of the foreman and assistants all had quit two to three weeks after I left, they lost very skilled labor they had kept there fifteen years or more walk out the door embarrassed, and feeling all confused and most likely made fun of, for mistakenly falling and having such feelings for another man, it hurt me to find all this out but I was not surprised, I had a feeling she wanted to call my bluff and not think I fooled anyone, and why not? I fooled her? Was this revenge? but I had to find another job, I am home maybe two weeks when I find a job working for a lab going out at night drawing blood from nursing homes a job that would be the hardest job I ever had to do and learn, but it was back to a woman's field 97 out of 100 employees would be female, and the hours where the worst, I got up at two in the morning was out by 4 am into the madness! what was I thinking, and then my oldest daughter needs to save money she asks if I would baby sit her son, if I do the six hundred she pays for day care each week she will give me half. It will help her with bills and me too so I say ok but am I going to be sorry I did that. A work week that should be 8 hour days turn into 12-13 hour days, with

8-9 hours pay no holidays but three a year, forget Christmas you just started, my daughter suddenly stops paying me, she said well why should I? All he does is sit and watch television. I said! oh really, What about me running to get him before 6 PM. or you get charged 15 dollars every minute I am late, and I just make it with my schedule, Then with him in the car I got take him with me shopping, get him back to the house cook his and everyone else's dinner, get myself ready for bed if I am lucky I will get 4-5 hours' sleep And then start all over again, are you kidding me? I tell her no! not any more find someone Else, so what does she do, drops him off at the house and takes off, leaving him standing at my door, this is horrible and just the beginning of how she will use and abuse me for the next ten years while I raise her kid for her. As she makes piles of money spends it only on herself, there were times she dropped him off so late I had to share my dinner with him, there was nothing to give him I would tell her but it went in one ear and out the next, this will be one of the reasons our relation has to end, she is a lousy mother, a disgrace, how could a mother do that, and one brought up so good she had everything, and a good home, we never left our kids with anyone, we took care of them ourselves, the very first time we went camping with our first baby she must have been 8-9 months and we got a good buzz on at the campsite but as we looked at our baby sleeping so innocent in her little car bed We realized if there was an accident or an emergency, We would not be in the right mind to drive or do the right things and something bad would or may result because we are to stoned, and we gave it up, the party was over for us we put all our effort into our children and protected them, Years later after, admitting she did bang her head that day and got me arrested, she would tell me her boyfriend would gag her, and tie his shirt around his fist and beat her unconscious she could scream for help and no one heard a thing, it also left no marks, this guy was a professional woman beater, a coward and a cheap thug. he also told her if she went to the police he would put a bomb under her parents car and when they went shopping he would blow up the car and kill her entire family, even her little sisters, she believed him, she was caught up in a cycle of abuse woman get in, He may have carried that out, who knows, I don't think so myself I believe he was nothing but a coward, He was a man who could rob eighty year old woman on the street with a knife. and just cut off their jewelry, Cut away the precious memories of their loved ones as they shook and trembled with fear, she was told do some for him but refused, I wish she went to the police and turned him in, it was true about the armed robbery arrest, and she knew, I believe she was an accomplice at this point, and she did nothing to help, those poor people from being robbed, I don't if she was attracted to the bad boy or just got in too deep and was afraid to get out, I know men and boys do and find themselves also into deep, I was almost into deep, but I got away from it, I didn't want to go too far, you can go underground if you want there is another world there, but that world is a darker world with lots of shadows and has no god and no god means no hope, no luck, no prayer, nothing to save you when the guy you work for thinks you betrayed him, he will tell you himself before he kills you god is not here to save you today, In California I had many offers to carry packages, I would not be told what's inside just deliver it, I met lots of gypsies and foreigners, there was good money in it, I would get my own gun for protection and if I got caught would get protection in jail. As long as I didn't snitch, I had an initiation where that I would have to prove I could do it, I would have to rob a store or gas station, break in a house just once to convince them I am not a cop and I can handle it, I was broke and I needed money, what an easy way to get it, but I always said no thanks, I will just get along my own way thanks for the offer, I never took that step, and I am so glad I never did, and I still always had a safe place to go in my mind when I got scared or frightened, and lonely, It was my happy place! I went when my dad beat me after work, or was scared about school the next day, I went there to ease the pain and heal, I developed it at a young age the first time I dressed as a girl I was seven years old, I was in the attic some neighbors from the old neighborhood from worlds end Hingham also moved, we stored some of their belongings in our attic. I got curios to what was in those boxes one day and I open up a box full of dresses, In my size they must have been there daughters, thing she must have grown out of, there was a large full length mirror attached to the wall big enough for two grownups, I went and got my mom's red lip stick, she always had that bright red lip stick that they all wore in the 60's and some blush. It's all I really knew about makeup as I watched my mom apply hers, and mascara a little tricky at first but you learn. That first time I saw myself in the mirror it was her, me, I felt real good, and alive, she was someone I really wanted to share with everyone it felt right but also very wrong. my feelings where so mixed I could see someone I always wanted to be, and share, but I was also scared I would get caught, why?

My little excursions where short lived, Minutes most of them, I just wanted to see her, I kept an image of her in my head to remember her, she was like a secret friend, I put her in a little box to hide and protect her, and I would often daydream and be playing with her inside our secret little box, as I grew older the box changed, it became nicer looking I turned it into a nice little jewelry box, also, I! changed from a little girl into a woman with nicer clothes, longer hair, we grew together, I felt safe, it's like I was locking myself safely away from harm, the real me safe in this tiny little box, safely playing and growing, becoming a woman while the outside that was a man looked for an identity to survive in as a male in the real world I really had to live in, One day working as a tool and die maker at a factory I had to go to the assembly lines to fix some broken tools and equipment and find out why they are breaking, a long work bench with about 20 people and machinery used to assemble the products, many of them where Asian and spoke little English. I had to communicate with them and also everything I did, and they did had to be written down, So I helped all of these people mostly woman, learn to speak better English and I corrected there spelling and sentence structure on their work sheets, so everyone knew what we were talking about and the reports that went into the office went smoother, something I found again I had to improve on myself writing this book so long after, The company had a tutor come in a couple hours a week but I gave them that extra one on one help they needed and they befriended me, they would even stop me in the hall and ask for help with a sentence or a word, and how to say it right, when they left after several months most where temps and worked on contracts, They came to me and gave me a gift I was not even expecting one.

It was a small tin ornate box, I open the box, it's plays music, it's a little jewelry box, inside there is a round mirror, also inside a small ballerina doll, I pick it up and put it on the mirror and it dances and twirls all around on the mirror like a sheet of ice, I feel like I am falling through the floor like an out of body feeling, just like when I went to the bus stop in kindergarten, I am holding in my hand what I once held in my mind, and was right there looking at it, what a feeling of being here before, how beautiful a gift, I still have it, I keep it locked away safe in a fireproof safe at home, I let no one touch it but me, and when

I have a really bad day I will take it out and open the box to let her out and dance on her little glass stage surrounded by red velvet, it's not exactly as the one I pictured in my mind, but it was so close spiritually, and I always wonder why they gave me such a gift, I was a man, I even had a beard, it may have been something they were selling and had a lot of or it may have been for someone else who did not show up for work that day, I will never know, I am just happy to have it, I am to someday be that woman that was locked in the box so many years waiting to be free, to really come out of that box forever and never have to go back in. I am now starting my new job at the lab; my youngest daughter has a boyfriend who stays at the house a lot. They eventually elope, no one knows for months they are married, that hurt me, I thought she would tell me anything she always did, He joined the army and just before he left they eloped. He was an Irish boy with a real love for his liquor, his whole family except his father a strict police officer, this boy could put down a case of beer and look sober as a priest, and I would run into him almost every night at 3 AM. in the morning getting ready for work, It never seemed to bother him that I was dressed as a woman on my way to work, he always said have a good night at work the hours where lousy but I had my privacy, I could come and go as I pleased, and now my youngest daughter has moved to Tennessee to join her army husband and soon I would get calls he was starting to abuse her, take her money, be gone on training missions for weeks and leave her without food, I would wire her money, she got caught DUI, driving him home she was only twenty, it was not that she was drunk it was the fact she was drinking, underage her level for the alcohol test was.02 to be drunk it's .08 I had to send her money I was saving for other things but it went to help her out of trouble. In a year I sent 5000 dollars, I had in my 401k she came back home and finally divorced him, I was still working, but my health was catching up to me, I liked what I was doing, it was a job caring for people it's not that I just went around to jab a needle into some poor sick dying elderly person, but it was watching the ends of many life's and those so frightened at the end, afraid where they were going from here, I always just looked at them and said, just keep your faith, I never said any name of any god or brought up any religion. I just said it as nicely and comfortably to them as I could and smiled, and told them they would be ok, they did not know nor did I ever tell any of them what I had seen as a child, the little girl who just floated over me and watched me sleep, I will never know where she came from, still I wake up at night and look to see if she is there, but I know these people leaving us now in this time of their life are going someplace, some people and therapist's I have mentioned this to say that I saw myself in a dream, that the little girl I saw, was me, myself, an hallucination from a dream, because I wanted to be a girl so bad, and they could almost convince me, Except for one thing, My sister saw her too, and I got to bring comfort to those who had no one left in their lives there friends and family where gone, Imagine being so lonely your happy to see someone about to jab you with a needle, and the care is not so good for a lot of them, from the richest homes to the poorest, the care was the same, all aids who cannot speak English frighten the patients, and nurses who went to college now won't get their hands dirty, the biggest surprise to me was patients that fell right by nurses who stood there yelling for the aid at the end of the hall, they would have to drop there blankets and towels and run as fast as they could to catch the patient before they fell, many never made it, 99 out of 100 of patients fell, when a nurse could have stepped a few feet in and prevented that from happening, I guess they did not want to hurt their back, Let someone who did not go to college do that, and these where woman, where and how and why did they lose their compassion, it's if the more power they had the meaner they got, just like men but they did not handle their authority right, they used it to make you subservient to them. They relish there power that they get, many don't get it and the few that do act it out wrong, like me learning and trying to be a man, I screwed up all the time, and I kind of knew what they felt like, I was learning that as living as a woman and being around them, not all where all into their emotions and feelings, somewhere abrupt and rude as men were, They tear each other apart with horrible gossip, when I was first around them and one would start to cry, I would panic, but all the woman around just looked on or ignored it. It was so confusing to me, they wondered why I would be so concerned too, it wasn't until I really got so deep in my own feelings as a woman and cried so much myself that I realized crying was so much a part of their life style that they don't react the way a man does when he sees a woman cry, in-fact it was almost a giveaway something was up with me, why was "I" so concerned, Men also gossip real bad worse than woman. But woman make most of it up, and they say what they suspect before they really know, men out right like to catch you in a weak moment then rip you up, But if they fist fight later have a beer it's over, woman hold grudges longer, these things where surprising to me, there are differences subtle little ones in between the big ones, it would sometimes give me a feeling of why go through all this if I am joining a gender that is not what I thought it was, my first idea that in becoming a woman I was becoming a part of the team, a team that brought most of what humanity needed, love and nurturing, but not all woman had that in them, And was all this worth it to be a part of this gender, I think so, I know one thing is, I live in one area of the world and it may be different all over, so I speculate a lot, but also go by what I have seen myself, even thinking back when I first came out at the first job, many where happy to accept me at first, it was false information and lies from a few bad people that scared them not me, and I myself have issues I am not what a man should be, so I realize there are all different steps in all genders, I have shown pictures of my old self to girlfriends I get to trust and they are just about drooling over my old self and I can't see why, I see an ugly guy with nothing, I don't even remember who he was, and in society I took a step down and had removed my "crown" as it was a man's world and I learned that so much working, the pay is not equal and the attitude towards a woman doing a man's job like I had done was unheard of, like when I was a child my mom and her neighbor friend had to hide when they smoked, woman back then would be called a bad woman if caught smoking in public, I saw signs on bar room doors that said men only, no woman allowed, at a young age I could see I was entering a man's world, and I was supposed to be one of them, take my place and glide right into it, but I resisted, it was not my world, I look at pictures now of groups of men in their suits from wedding parties or office clubs, I am so glad I don't look like them, I have no desire to ever in my life put on a three piece suit again although I notice men get distinguished with age while woman dry up and wither like fruit once firm and ripe now wrinkled and withdrawn, But I would still be happier to look like one, It's not so much the look of old age it is the years of nurturing their souls that is important, Inside the ones who have become what they were born to become, And embraced there femininity, they are the ones who can still look at you and give you that warm smile knowing all too well the beauty of their youth has gone, but you can tell their souls have grown and the beauty from the outside has gone inward and has gone deep into their souls so deep they feel your pain without you saying a word, that is the journey into womanhood I love the most, men can and do get in touch with their emotions but society will only let them go so far, to cry out in public as a man is an embarrassment, may as well put on a dress, and when I tried hard to be one pushing away those feelings, it left a feeling of emptiness and also if I showed any emotions at all I was weak, It was safer for me to be who I am in this lifetime as a woman, I am very soft with my touch and kind, very sensitive and very emotional. I don't belong in a male's body. What I wear for clothing is an expression of my feelings and I am showing everyone who it is I am that I want to share, as much as it is the sign of being a woman, the clothing we wear that separate' our genders to me is important, It shows who each of us we are, it also helps us determine the human we are looking at, is the suitable mate for baring children, and producing off spring And the continuation of life, and I believe we should always have a dress code of some type, We should not all wear just what we want out and around the planet not knowing who is who, I love that difference, it's very important, and it's all over in nature everywhere you look, what I have gone through I would never wish on my worst enemy, but to really look into my own heart and to feel I can be myself and express my feelings in this world then I must dawn the clothing of a woman, I have already lived half my life as a man and half as a woman and never want to go back, it was a journey into my soul I never could have imagined. My doctors told me I would change physically which of course I wanted, but they said there would be emotional ones also, I would be more sensitive and learning to deal with an increase of all my emotions excluding anger, was so much more than I ever imagined, I don't know if every woman feels like this, It maybe that I went in search of it, I wanted to find and embrace it as if it where the treasure I imagined it would be, and it became a search so deep into my soul that after finding and feeling who I was really inside I never would want to be anyone else. It was a treasure more wonderful than I ever imagined, I can wonder that if I was born so lucky. to physically come out correct whether or not I would have just took it for granted as some woman do and I don't believe I would have, I am still me, and my search was not so much a search to become a woman, but to search my soul to see if I could or would be good enough to have such an honor to be called a woman, From what is coming from my heart and mind and not what I looked like on the outside, and I did find it.

I did find that I don't need dresses and make up to make me feel I can be a woman now, it's always been there, it needed to grow and be nurtured to mature, The clothing is just one of the wonderful parts of it I get to enjoy, and when I see my own self I recognize myself at once, as the woman I have become and want to share with everyone else who wants to embrace me, and I do my best to show that my journey to become myself was not one in vain or a selfish one but it was a journey I want to share, not by so much looking the part but by really being the part, and I have succeeded, I will keep moving forward without any regrets, And never look back, and prove that I made the right choice with as many acts of kindness I can give out, and I will always be inside my soul looking for more love and understanding and if I make mistakes work hard to correct them, find and embrace what makes us who and what we are, my search will never end, as I will always look to perfect myself as the woman I want to become as long as I live, I know I can keep doing better, as I have gone into a journey, Not as so much a journey to find out who I am but to learn to love who I have become, that was the hardest part, with all the negativity the world and the people in my life around me have thrown at me to give up and abandon this journey have all failed. It was too important to me not to give up on myself, And not be who and what they want me to be anymore, there the selfish ones not me, but they would want me to commit suicide and be the ones who said it was me doing a selfish act, but I still have a way to go, while working at the lab I have another mild stroke and the hours and shifts are very stress full along with caring for a child that's not mine I get CIDP it is an auto immune disorder.

My immune system is now attacking my body, the coating that covers my nerves is being eaten away by a dominant protein I have had Charcot Marie Tooth disease and a lot of arthritis from many back injuries. One they say is congenital, or happened very early in life. My mother told me she had to chase me to the bus stop every morning to kindergarten at Hingham when I was four, with a hair brush and smack my behind, I remember that, it hurt like hell and it was not that I hated going to school it was when I got to the bus stop and noticed the difference in clothes that boys and girls wore I felt out of place, I was scared, I felt like I would leave my body every time I looked at the girls who huddled together and watched me join the crowd. And the snicker on boys faces as they too watched me as if they all knew, I wanted to be a girl but was not allowed to be one, and I was right about that, when I ran into that kid from the old neighborhood in worlds end in high school, who told me that when I was between 2-4 years old they would all come down to my house and catch me outside and beat me, because I was the little boy who wanted to be a girl, seemed like everyone who wanted to hurt me, did, I wonder if they or my mother caused the injuries to my lower back that I now suffer horrible pain from. And it made working very hard, driving all day hitting bumps, I could feel electric shocks hitting my brain in waves, that would intensify as the day wore on, I was taking up to 15-20 nitroglycerin tablets a day at times to stop the angina attacks I was having as I walked up to the nursing homes to draw blood, I would pop nitro—like candy to get through the day, and my doctor said with my tiny artery condition and spasms it is ok to take when I needed to But my schedule was bad for me, as with most people the rule is by the third one you better be at a hospital, once I had an attack that was so bad it took thirteen hours to get the monitors at the hospital I was at to read normal, I really thought that day was my last, I got to a point that all the fear came and reached a peak I was so frightened it felt like I had high voltage electricity running all through me. Sticking into me like sharp pins just like someone ran me underneath a sewing machine at super high speed, the bed felt like it was shaking, and then all of a sudden calm. All the fear and pain left and I felt so peaceful. The nurse came in and checked me I had nitroglycerin paste all over me, It looks like the glue you make in kindergarten to glue paper things together, there was always a few kids that ate it, she asked how I felt and I said I felt so relaxed and peaceful I said I never ever felt so at peace, I said what did you give me something good, but she looked at the heart monitor and back at me and looked scared, as if she had seen that peaceful look before, maybe in people about to die, who's fear had gone away and they felt it was time to let go, and I really believe I got that far, I was that close to dying, but I recovered she put paste all over me and put more nitroglycerin under my tongue I stayed in the hospital three days and was finally cleared to be sent home, but I had become so exhausted and my auto immune really flared up bad after an EMG test, I could barely walk I looked awkward walking I could not feel my leg's I just threw them out and hoped I would land on them and not fall. The lab wanted to put me on disability and send me home permanently, As I am waiting to be discharged I am saying good bye to some friends I made at work A woman comes out and asks will you work here for me? Please it's desk job oh please I want you to work for me, let me show you what you will do, she pushed me into the building on a chair with rollers, everyone was afraid I would fall, so I had to go in by chair, I was so surprised I never met her before and new nothing about her, I had no idea why she picked me, was this a horrible job or something,? But it wasn't too bad it was a customer service job and I was so glad I took it. But I was going to have to talk on a phone all day and that was a scary, scary moment, I have come so far and not just with the sex change part of my growth but the fears all my life of interacting with people like in high school when I just froze walking into the building when teachers and other students, "kids" when I think back now, all looking at me, I froze like a deer in headlights. and was terrified about what to say to a girl once I got close or try to build a relationship with her, even a neighbor across from my grandmother's house in Hingham I knew since I was about ten when I went over to do chores, we hung out a lot when we became teens and smoked pot together in the playground where we once played on the swings and slides, and still even with her I can't open up, She always asks what are you thinking about, you never talk, you just think all the time, tell me what it is, I tell her I just like to think in my mind that I am free! That's all. that's all I could think of I was just too scared to tell her what I was thinking as I traveled along with my secret friend, If anyone knows what crying as a teenager is I do, I those three pillow three pillows! I used to soak wet, And when they told me taking hormones where going to make me cry more and I would more sensitive, I didn't think anyone else but god knows and feels for you when you cry like that, If he is busy with the world's problems I know I cried deep enough and often enough for him to hear me, I don't know if he will forgive me for believing, or even thinking I was born a woman in a man's body, I don't know if this is some trial or test he put me through, I hope my tears prove my soul is in pain and not trying to just please itself for its own vanity and that I love myself more than I love god, and I talk about my beliefs in god a lot I honestly believe we are here for all of his trials and test, but I rarely go to any church, I spend so much of my time in self prayer for help so often as it is, that when I go and sit in a church and relax, I just feel a chill or a rush of tingling up my back then throughout my body, it feels like I am being lifted off the bench, I get in this feeling and I don't want to participate in the kneeling and standing and singing and the joining in of the ceremonies inside with all the people, if I do I lose my connection and the routine of the churches become boring and I find that no matter what type of church I go to eventually I must reflect the majority of the followers and become just like them or not really be accepted, just like in real life like my gender identity issue among people who know who I was before or what I have done to be where I am today, and I can't be like them, I don't fit in their view of the world's opinion of who I should be, they to judge me, and most are not very kind, So what I do here is between me and god only, not anyone else, and I only hope is that I have come here and have succeeded in what he had planned for me to do, all the many little things or maybe one big one in the end, And what puzzles me now is why did this woman want me to work for her, I thought I did a terrible job as a phlebotomist It was one of the hardest jobs I ever had to learn Especially on old sick, dying bruised dehydrated people many who hated it, and fought back with scratches, kicks, punches, bites, pulling hair, and spitting, and now I had to talk to customers on a phone, with this ugly male voice of mine, I got into many fights growing up, my nose got hit a lot and I ended up with a real low nasal voice like someone pinched my nose when I talked, I have hated my entire life, by sight ok but on the phone. No! that's bad, I know they were suspicious already I had to call in so much to communicate, but no one said anything, the only sticky part at any job was always Providing health insurance as a family plan, it always meant I had to confess. Insurance won't cover same couple relationships, I did not want to any give it away anymore I felt she should get her own at her job, but I did, I was always the provider and was the one who got the health insurance for the family, I went into personal and told the woman in personal, about where I was and that I was eligible for the family plan with another woman on my plan I had special circumstances and the laws are correct because we married as a traditional couple and did not divorce so we still remain married, We were one of the few two woman maybe the only filing tax returns jointly before they even changed the marriage laws, federal and state laws also, we are legally married and she is entitled to all my benefits, She treated me better than anyone in the past ever in human resources, and I had completely fooled her, she loved it, she got such a kick out of me coming in and telling her, we were always good friends after that I showed her some old pictures of myself, she would just laugh, she was fun to talk with, she rode a big Harley and you would never know, she was so sweet looking, she fooled me too, I read up on how woman talk differently, I learned they talk with their mouths and not their throats and use there tongue more so I practiced real hard, but it was while at work, I would hear someone say a customer wants to speak to the man they just spoke too, and say what man? There are no men here, I wanted to die, it went on for a while, and I just pulled into my cubicle and hid, but I kept going, it took a year but soon I was getting a lot of yes miss, thanks miss, at work and at home. I was surprised, it was working, I heard my self-played back on a recording once and for the first time I did not recognize my own voice, it startled me then just filled me with relief, and joy I had done it. And what really began to surprise me was the confidence I had as a woman I was no longer frightened to walk by people or into crowds, I have a walk of confidence, I developed a very confident female walk, not flamboyant just a nice confident swing to my body that felt like me. And I can talk openly in front of people when at one time I just hid in the corner, afraid to speak at all, These changes where ones I never expected, I thought I would be a shy timid girl at best, but I have become the opposite, I am stronger and braver than I have ever been before, and I keep going along this is so right, and I know now if I got to wear a nice pretty dress to kindergarten as a child my mother would not have had to chase me there with a hair brush, I would have been an all "A" student I am sure, with lots of friends, And had a lot more potential than that depressed little boy I was, sitting alone all day dreaming of either being the girl who I really wanted to be, or planning a suicide. A few months go by and father's day weekend is about to arrive, and I get an email from my boss, do you still celebrate?

I went blank, and got a cold chill right up my back, like a cold wave hit me, she knew! And if she does, how many other people in here do? I write back, you knew about me? But I bet before the email was at her computer I was in her office. She was just smiling all over. Of course I know, I am your boss they told me, The minute I found that out, I had to have you work for me, I think you are so awesome, She told me that when she was a little girl, Her mommy died. And that her dad took care of the family and he played both rolls to make us happy, and brought us up the best he could, we were dirt poor but we all loved each other. My dad was there, he kept us all together and did his best to make sure we had everything we needed, I was so honored that she related me to someone as close to her as her father, it didn't matter it was a male figure just the admiration alone was one of the nicest compliments of my life, going into this new one. after the weekend I got to my desk at work and wrote back, by the way, I had an awesome weekend, she yelled back this time as our cubicles where all in tight and close, too bad you can't share that can you? I said no! I brought in a couple of the cards my kids gave me, and showed them to her privately in her office, each card with dad on it. My kids still call me dad I found there are some things I have compromise's on as I go along and also there is only so much you can take away from your children, as long as when I die they bury me in a nice dress, invite everyone to my funeral. Make sure Cynthia's friends get a chance to say goodbye it would not be right if they did not, But I told them they can just write a large DAD on my stone, no names, Just my birth date if they want, all their friends always called me that to, doesn't matter who, but once they get to know me, Whoever they hung with would call me dad, it is a name that always just sticks with me, like more of a nick name, I remember when I used to pick up my grandson and shop for groceries after work, once going through the checkout aisle the woman says thank you miss. And my grandson gets real angry and says that's no miss that's my grand dad, she just looked shocked! she looked back at me, back at him, back at me, with her hands on her face, I was so embarrassed, I shop there all the time, now I was going to be scared to, I pulled him aside and told him not to speak to people like that! It is not polite! And when someone makes a mistake like that it's rude to correct them! Don't ever do that again! If it doesn't bother me, it shouldn't bother you, people make mistakes and should not get yelled at every time they did, he said ok, never had that happen again I got a lot of thank you misses and a little grin out of my grandson, He was five, now I had a feeling now I was going to be raising a son, this I never thought out, I wondered how that would be, one thing I found is you can certainly break the heart of daddies little girls doing what I have done, you can only hope the love you gave will be returned someday, and I know a boy would be crushed if his dad went and decided to become a woman, it would have been just as hard maybe harder but either way a different set of problems, And my grandson was all boy, and I would never influence a boy in any way to act out as a girl, I myself would not even hand him a doll to play with unless he wanted to play with it himself; if he had one I would not take it away and make him feel bad or punish or humiliate him either, it would only be bad, I would never want to see any child go through this, knowing how I felt even as a small child; if I saw a small child like myself, especially a boy, my heart would just break, I know what he is in for, and I would hope now his chances will be better than mine where, once my grandson brought a pink marshmallow fluff sandwich to school, and came home all upset, He said don't you ever give me a girly sandwich again ever to bring to school, the kids picked on me all day, Things have not changed much, My biggest and worst fear is someday coming out my front door I will be shot dead by someone who thinks he is doing the world a favor and my second is it will be my oldest daughter behind the trigger claiming she did the family a favor, or if not the trigger man in-advertly say something to a killer in a bar that's comes out some night looking for blood, that my kind will only breed others like myself, and they would feel emasculated, and my feelings are, woman are better off with a male like myself, one hundred years ago or five hundred to a thousand, yes maybe then woman needed that male warrior, to be there, but now with technology and the advances in civilization, men are losing their place, their foot hold on being the king, woman are now more selfsufficient and provide for themselves, but still require a male to produce off spring, a male like myself accepted in the environment and adored by woman as a suitable mate would be very good, I myself would care for the babies as much maybe even more, my life is proof enough that I have thought more of my children and gave them opportunities to evolve and grow, while I sat back waiting for my turn, just like at dinner I cooked every ones meal and made sure every child had enough to eat before I had my own, and one thing I always still do to remember my grandmother, is I always wash my own plate after I eat my meal, I did mine for her, she was older and tired and if she was to tired I did all the dishes if she let me, but I always washed mine for her, and to this day since a child and at the time I lived with her I still do, my wife's comfort and care would also be a concern to me that she was always happy and was in love with me and wanted me there for those special needs from tender touches of romance to a nice warm bubble bath I would be so happy to give her, and I believe the male who wants to always dominate woman and see that they never want to choose a male like myself would go as far as killing us, and that what brings us to where I am in need of a gender reassignment surgery to fit in and have that part of my life very private, but my oldest daughter took my privacy away upon the very first day I moved into my home, I will have to eventually leave here to ever feel safe again, so careful you parents out there making your boys lunch leave out the pink fluff the worlds not ready for that yet, another thing that happens to me comes as a sad moment, I was planning on visiting the mother of my old childhood friend from hull, one I met at the age of seven, and still know till this day, I wanted her to know what I was doing and where I was in my life, she was always a person who traveled the city, In search of the best doctors and specialists for her kids, she taught me how to ride the subways into where all the really good hospitals where, she always said if you got anything you need to find out about yourself that's where to go, and she was right, I found my best resources on the same routes I traveled many times with her and my mother into the city, and I learned a lot about how to get around in town, I would often see her in my travels as a teen in the train stations as we exchanged trains we always waived, sometimes I gave her a ride home from Quincy square, where I would park my car, the hardest part at the time was deciding what to wear, a dress or just slacks, I was deciding on the dress, that first impression means the most, and I looked forward to revealing myself to her, I really felt that I would not have surprised her at too much at all, I always got little hints dropped at me from my mother, one was a talk show program with the subject of transgender on it, my mom told me hey, I think there is a show you might be interested in watching, when I walked into the television room I was shocked She sent me in to watch a show like that, and on a program like that it was Jerry Springer type show. I walked right out, not mad, just so surprised, it was that, she does know something feeling again, and what's she hiding. Also when I ran into an old friend again from worlds end Hingham, This time a girl I knew, my mother got a call from her mother and she said she was so happy and hoped I would be back to see her daughter again, and I was happy too, She was very cute and pretty, and both our parents where happy about this, I wondered why, my mom usually hates any relationships I get into, or my sisters (she gets involved) Then she throws in! Her mother is concerned she has a similar problem like you! I thought what problem? What is she telling me, what's she really hinting at here? I do see her again she is a very pretty girl and I am curious. She is 16 and I am 16 also we were neighbors once, and went to school together, I find her and we talk casually, and along comes her girlfriend, she pulls her aside and they talk, looks like a little fight, she comes back, and says I need to go I promised her we would do something today, again I try and the same girl again shows up and keeps her distracted. And keeps her far away as they talk, I feel something is not right, and I feel rejected so I give it up after four attempts, every time I try to visit, her friend comes over and takes her away, later I find they are lovers from a friend at school, I am all of a sudden embarrassed, what the hell is my mom thinking, The other thing is the mother of my friend I grew up with from hull was also at one time best of friends with my mother, And that's why I felt she would not be to surprised, it seemed she was in her way trying to help me back then with the trains and finding doctors in the city, all of a sudden one night as I am just coming in from work my wife tells me there was a fire in a house in hull and a woman died in it, an elderly woman and she read the address, I check, it's her, I am in shock I was about 6 to 8 weeks from a visit I had planned, I get a call from one of her sons he had heard I changed my name, and found me in the phone book, I said I had, but I said that I did not want to come down dressed up to a crowd I haven't seen in so long and I felt I need to tell my best friend first then let him see me as a woman later and I did not want to take the spotlight it was not a day for me, and that I would try to look like my old self as much as possible, I wore all my old men's clothes dressed all in black and there was also the possibility I would meet someone else there someone who in my life I never forgot. And was very special to me and had a very special place still in my heart, a candle still lit and warm, I walk into the chapel entrance I see her with her husband and her mother, she had not changed a bit, she just took over presence of the room like many times before, It was her! My very first love! As radiant to me as ever, we have come across each other again, I say hello, I am an old friend of the family and she looks up, and said which one are you? I was a little surprised, but I have changed a lot, I have not been called sir in over five years and my once blonde hair was dark black, I turned to her mother and said what about you? remember me?, she says no (same thing) which one are you?, then it hit's me, they think I may be one of my sisters, there were four of them, and my two brothers where still very young, way back before we moved, I looked at her, I said it's me! we dated once, and her face dropped, the look of surprise was all over her, I got that beautiful smile I loved to see again once more and a big hug, she introduced me to her husband and off I went, I saw my old friend way up front with his girlfriend I stayed in the back and listened to the sermon, And we went over to one of the sons homes to have a lunch, and talk about old times. I noticed. I was looked at a lot and I heard people ask who that woman is. I forgot about those breasts I can't really hide those anymore, sports bras do help but I have grown out of that now, that doesn't help much anymore, and my face has become very feminine looking, I sit and talk to some people on a rear deck where I find her, I sit and say hi, how have you been, she said good how about you? I said fine, we just made small talk, I made fun of her not recognizing me but she said the black hair fooled her the most, Before I left I got her email and gave her mine, it had a female name on it. She looked at it funny, then I said take this one too it's my own private one, she said ok, my first email was the truth the other I had to go home and hope I could get, someone could already have it, We emailed for days, as I explained myself she listened well, and very sincere but she also seemed relieved at what she may have had to have gone through if she had stayed with me, it seemed to frighten her, and was coming back to frighten me, I felt her fear, But I went into how there was such a different connection, with her and me, I can't say that if had stayed with her I would have taken it this far, but I would have tried a lot harder to work it out so both of us never would get hurt, and who I was married to now, never completely understood me and pushed that side of me away instead of nurturing me and growing together, I said I would like to come down to meet her family and she agreed, I wondered what she was thinking seeing me again as a woman and what was she explaining to her two daughters, She was meeting with an old boyfriend who was now a woman, and there was my feeling that I know as now as I write this book, she was the one!

she was that one back then that I loved so much, would I have done all of this? And sought out to change my gender so drastically, anything that would take away that sparkle in her eyes and the warm beautiful smile on her face that just says everything is ok, even when with all the exploring I have done? Those seemingly endless days of pains, and some experiences so wonderfully breathtaking I would never imagine, the journey into becoming a woman has been the most amazing experience I have ever placed myself in and I would say no, if I was still young enough to be saved! and always be that much in love, If she would have excepted the person who I kept hiding away was me, and if she loved me as much as I loved her I know she could have nurtured that part of me so that I myself would accept what I am and I would not take myself away from someone who loved me so much, and would have found a way to work it into our lives to a point clothing and makeup would have been the small details they are now, that is one thing I have learned so much about myself as I went on this journey alone. The clothing and makeup are the nicer parts of it. and it shows on the outside the person I am inside I want to share, anyone who loved me while still very, young could have nurtured me into a wonderful husband, and I do not believe I would wear feminine clothing or as least not as much to feel good about myself, Even my own wife may have been able to help back when I was very young although I was not in love, when we met I hoped for it to grow, and I have heard of it happening. I always give it time, it's time to root, sometimes it takes a long time to reach the surface, but I am patient there is too much in this lifetime for one soul to learn in its short time here. I have never given up, I just patiently wait for a decision, as my life comes closer to the end, I am still trying to this day hoping this day is a new one and it will get better from here, only at the beginning she did not want to nurture that part of me, once she shut me out and I got that part of me hurt. I could not feel it anymore, and I shut her out also, I don't feel she is happy she married a woman, it hurt bad, to bruise my own soul, and make it lonely again, or have someone who knows what can hurt you the most and then say it, and at my weakest point, foreplay, if I get hurt or rejected during my most favorite intimate part of embracing, I will get hurt, scared and back away real fast, it is the worst time to feel rejection and I never go there anymore, it terrifies me, and the emptiness afterwards, it's like the loneliness of an echo you hear bounce off a mountain then slowly fade away into silence as it disappears into nothing, the blanket wrapped around my body keeping me warm in death fantasies all the time, and still even though I had come so far, no one came with me, as if I got on the train all by myself went through scary tunnels and high hills and saw some beautiful scenery, and stormy days, met some friendly passengers and some that would kill and rob me, What a ride to take, friends and people come with you but the further down the track you go some get off and the train empties, The ones that love you the most stay on the longest, but the train pretty much empties out, but the one who love you the most they sit right up front with you helping you with the dark scary tunnels coming down steep scary hills, And those drops that suddenly come when you are driving ahead without a bump in so long, you think they have all come along, but when you get off at the station to take a break and look for them, a lot of them are not there, you just stand there alone looking down the empty dark track hoping there on the next train coming, hoping that someday they will get on it and come and join you, the loneliness society puts someone like me in is horrible, it is so bad, that just that one time I got a chance to fall in love and be happy, I never wanted to let go of what that felt like, it was so important that I did, when the world just beats you down every day for this, it is so hard to feel anything good, so many people are forcing me back and it so hard to, and it will have consequences, if you go back you can have a mastectomy to have your breasts and removed, but there will be scars, your hair grows back on your legs, back, and chest along with your urges to have sex again. I went off hormones almost 9 months once in between doctors. I swear I was going through male puberty again all over, I never watch porn or look at anything that might arouse me, I have completely shut myself off from any form of love even to love myself, I don't really feel my wife excepts me being a woman, she tried in the beginning but I really see it in her eyes, that she does not, and I really need to feel like somebody loves me before I can really embrace them, it's very hard now, it's not like when I was young and very powerful and I could go all night, Viagra, I never would have needed it, I still have some to spare to that guy and a few of his friends, even with the male hormone blocks It took it a long time to stop my erections especially to wake up with them, but peeing got rid of them, I just hate them, it's feeling so much like a man and also I feel a lot of "power" in my mind when that happens a power that made me feel I want to dominate my mate and be in control, what an awful feeling to me it was, It was my chemicals from being aroused and having male hormones take over, I do not want that at all, I looked once in my doctors folder who is adjusting my hormones when he was out of the office for a moment, I did nothing wrong they are my own records, under Cc, for chief complaint it reads, erections especially in am, method of treatment work with medication to ease patients anxiety, thank you doc, how many times in my mind I took out an old straight razor and just cut it off and I knew that's why I could not have had a male lover while I still have one, if aroused I to may also want to dominate, it is the chemicals released in my brain it's normal, I don't want to chance it, and I am sure another male lover is interested in my penis and I am not, and what is so good for me now is the blocks that I take, have taken that feel to dominate away, I have no urges to feel that feeling of overpowering anymore and I like that it's gone But I know if a woman who I am in love with wants me it won't be a dominating feeling now as much with all the changes I have been through It will be me surrendering for her and accepting me as I am now I am not looking for a feeling to dominate, if I do not have my surgery and I would still get aroused the feelings to dominate would not be there as much with a woman, and any woman that will someday allow me to have her would only feel to me a gift of love and not anything more, I am someone stuck in the middle that no one really wants, and I feel it all around me, only a woman would ever have the patience I will now need to allow me to cry away the fear of not scaring her away, With the gentle touch of my hands like it has happened before, and I cannot handle such a rejection again even once more in my life, I would die, I have been so alone so long and so afraid now of interacting I have kept myself away and denied any love or affection, for over twenty years now, not a good thing to do, I don't recommend it, get help young and early, as for myself I cannot handle any more rejection especially something so intimate, it would be the end, I would warn no one and just leave, I hear a little joke now and then, when you get that new sport car in the driveway aren't you taking it for a test drive? but we will see about that, I am getting too old and I don't expect it, and the love and nurturing that I have received all my life has been from woman, the change would be very life changing And maybe unwanted by any man, by him or myself and if it was a man he would really have to be someone very, very special to my heart, or it would not be any good for myself as I want to embrace every emotion of the moment I want to feel every part of what I am as a woman and can give and let myself go, it is so hard to say I can change now but also they say after surgery there is another big change emotionally and I have to believe them, they haven't lied yet, about these emotional shifts, but I do not think a man will ever reach this heart now, it has traveled to far inside, And now I am going to visit this family for the first time, and I decided on the dress I was too wear the same one I picked out to meet her aunt in, I met them all and we had taco's for dinner, they were all nice sweet girls not shy to talk to me, I stayed about two hours, they showed me a movie of their wedding, I held back tears through the entire movie, once I saw her in that bridal gown it hit me so hard, there she was walking down the aisle with her man, She was as beautiful as a bride as I always imagined her, and here I am sitting with a dress on watching it, What a place I took, it's if I just stepped aside slipped into a dress and let a real man take my place. and walk down the aisle with the only woman in my life I was ever in love with, never in my lifetime had I ever felt that again ever, just came once, I tried hard to grow it, nurture it, to say I do, and will, but the feel of it was never the same, it's like it's always a jar little empty never will fill all the way, no matter how much you put in, you can't even fill it enough to reach in and touch it or feel it. I emailed later, I wondered what her kids thought of me, she said they loved me, and especially they both loved my shoes, I was happy about that, my shoes of all things, It is the one thing I am so picky about and have so much trouble finding, and one of my most favorite accessories, I have such bad feet from the CMT. It makes your arch very high. To get a compliment on my shoes was the best, I knew I was going to like her daughters very much, and one of them I that I would get to know more, as time went on has become so close in my heart as if she was my own daughter, I share some of my little emotional stories with her, that she so patiently listens to, I may be boring the hell out of her but she is still so very kind to listen, And another most very important woman in my life that had been able to reach into my heart was my therapist, my depression was bad and my health was getting bad she was keeping me on that page of caring for myself, and not because she got a paycheck either, I knew she really cared, I had gotten to a point I could share anything, at first I thought why not, this is what she is there for, she is not really experienced in gender reassignment, and I know I may have gone into some of our sessions and really shocked and surprised her with the answers and problems I faced but I was not holding back, she had a real heart, it's what I needed, There could never be a better doctor patient relationship ever, if I ever lost her I would to be lost myself, she has become a very important woman in my life, I have feelings as strong as love, and that was good, even though she is a doctor. we always are professional I really have a feeling in my heart for her, and I need that, and went through some very wonderful little crushes on her I kept to myself, it was good to have feelings like that, she is another butterfly in my clutter, and I hoped someday, There might be a chance I will fall In love again even once more, and I will be so happy, I have not had feelings of being in love for so long, I told my therapist I had come across someone I once knew, that special one, you never get over, we all have, that special love, We carry with us to remind us what we once had so someday we may give it back again to the right person and never make any mistakes that would cause you to lose that wonderful moment that the person who loves you back, gives you. she was very happy that I had found something again as special to myself as that that and I could share myself as a new girlfriend to, and have a wonderful woman for a friend, to talk to so intimately to and hopefully someone who understands me enough to grow along with me and share my emotions and feelings as a woman as I am growing along into womanhood myself, she knows of my struggle at home with all the conflicts, of growing into a woman and the panic in the family, it just seemed to blow everything apart, and I was always running around with pieces of sting, glue, and tape, trying to keep it all together, Plus work these crazy hours and raise my grandson whose mother, my oldest daughter seemed to care so little about, she was just all for herself, riding expensive cars smashing them up drunk, getting another, leaving him with me all the time, it all caught up I kept getting auto immune flair ups and missed work too much, they had to let me go, social security read all my doctor reports and said stay home on a phone interview, I was shocked, what no work,? I was that bad, and they were right she tried for years to get me to admit it, but I kept going till it almost killed me, I had a couple weeks I was so exhausted and ready to go, I worried my children would find me dead soon, And my wife all she had to say was, you better have an income. I don't care what no money out you go, I am not supporting you, how she forgets when we started out and did not work the first ten years, I did, I took care of her the kids everything on my own, she only started part time ten years later, so she would feel it was her own spending money, I paid for everything, I just did it! I knew it was my responsibility at the time, And here I am sick with some serious health issues and she is mad now she is the one going to work, in a job she hates, nurses aid work, what a horrible job, no one but foreigners will do that now, the pay is so low and the work brakes your back because there are not enough staff, but that was her choice, she had many chances to change her career but never did, just complained a lot, it was like trying to get her to move to another apt, or get a different car, you just can't keep fixing them, and living in places bad for your children just because the rent is a little lower, and you have no car payment, you need to be where you are happy, but she is stubborn and won't let go almost like a hoarder, after her mom had that stroke all of this started to change her, she was not at all the girl I married, she had turned into someone else, people say it's me that did it to her, no! it was her that changed before Cynthia arrived years before, she will not change or except change, and one of those changes I really believe she cannot except is me, she won't say it, but it shows, She is depressed all the time complains repeatedly over the same issues daily, and keeps making the same mistakes, I know she was a deprived child, All her siblings were, excluding her older brother, her father seems to love his sons and grandsons but not to welcoming to his daughters and granddaughters, his sons visit all the time and her sister can come up and visit him from Florida, several times a year and stay a week, he knows she has money and won't need a buck or two but. He will only let her visit once a year, on her birthday, just before the holidays and he gives a card with two hundred dollars just after he tells her everything he hates about her and us and all her mistakes and she is nothing to him anymore she comes home crying every time she visits I have told her to just give it up. it's not worth the lousy 200 dollars he gives you, and what is so sad he always left out his granddaughters except once or twice, but never forgot his grandsons they all got a card with money in it too, mine got nothing, pictures of them where all over his house and none of my daughters, and I feel guilty a lot about it, it's my fault, I am feminine and it's a quality he does not like and considers useful only in a wife he can control, and on a Christmas day he slammed the door in their faces, it is a day none of us has forgotten and never will ever, I hope in his life's review on his judgment day that's one thing god show's him and asks why he did it, How cruel was that, to do that to little girls with smiling faces at your door on Christmas day to come and see you on Christmas morning, only a savage, a real monster And how could a woman who grew up without any love know what it is like to feel it, it has to be a very mixed feeling. And I feel deeply for her pain and I am still here with her, I am waiting patiently still for her to decide to let me back in to her heart again or not, and it has to be done in acts of faith, I have shown patience kindness and understanding now for almost twenty years, I think that is enough for any one, I know I don't feel I was ever loved as a child either it was all pretend love, and bribery. Feeling it again is hard I was never that boy they really wanted, I was rejected in the end for a stranger, and everything of my fathers was sold away, to strangers, one precious memory of my grandfather I loved so that everyone was afraid of but me, although at the beginning I was, he was in a mental hospital 20 years and I was told he had fits of rage, I was afraid at first, but he was very kind, you just had to reach him, all I ever felt was depression and rejection, my two most experienced feelings, it was the only real familiar feeling like I always had a nice warm blanket around me, like Charlie brown the comic with Linus and his blanket, it was a feeling sometimes I brought it up myself just so I could cry, but the thoughts that go along with it are horrible and nightmarish, not the wonderful tears you experience from love, and loss of loves, The economy in the late 2000's is real bad we tried to remortgage several times but it all went bad, the banks promised you money to do the repairs and pay off bills get that new car, but when you came to sign they said we need 6 months of steady payments to prove to us you can handle your mortgage, then we will give you that money, but 6 months later, it was sorry your credit score was not good enough. This happened several times in the meantime take thirty thousand off your equity, and in two years raise your interest so your payments get too high, and because you could not do repairs, can't sell. And have to try and refinance. and now I understand this housing crunch, for a few years the banks rolled us all around in a barrel then shook the money out of us leaving us dizzy were not the only ones lied to and left in a house you owe more than it's worth, the banks they have lost nothing don't be fooled they scammed the American people right out of their property, and the government and the first black American president who says he cares and will help. Bails out the banks and not the people I don't think he will repeat another term, it will be a miracle and another miracle if he gets it right the second time around, if not, I fear the end of this country is around the corner, and war is brewing, why would banks get money, they already did, they stuffed their pockets with every ones falsely raised equity, the stress of being short on money and all these changes and the effects on people around me are deepening the hole I am digging myself into of depression, it's like a roller coaster that keeps going deeper down and deeper and you never come back to the surface again ever, I should not be worrying about the world I need to worry about me, thoughts of killing myself are day long activities, I don't even hear what people are saying when they talk to me, I just drift off hoping I will be out of here someday, my hormone doctor leaves the hospital, And tells me to find a replacement where he is going they will not let him do the practice of helping transgender people, I feel I am lost. What do I do now, I don't want to start over and have those ups and down's and change back even a little, I try a local endocrinologist, who at first seems willing but then at the end backs away because I have already had strokes, but the strokes are not related to the hormones it was other factors, I am at a loss again I need to find another one or I will start going backwards again, And it's not good, it's dangerous for your health, and a possible life and cancer risk, I find a woman northern mass her name Dianne she is wonderful and very experienced this is her field, an expert, and a woman too, a real plus, if I can communicate how I feel to another woman, I feel even more to myself I am on the right path, and she herself also could read into me easier and more clearer and also know that we are being two females talking together in a room, she finds me another doctor, same hospital from before, he was the other doctors replacement, He stepped up to help all the people who got left behind when the other left, someone had to, I guess the line at the door was longer than they thought, and I was back again on my hormones and getting my levels adjusted, I am at this point not there, 90-10 0r 900 to 100 parts per, for the female spectrum I was lagging behind, my female was high but my male was to and that is a stroke risk, But I am older this time and given less Premarin and more of a male block for health reasons, so it took a long time to adjust my levels and the time it took I have PMS's so bad and along with the depression and everything going on at my house that suicide. Was really becoming what I thought was the only way to stop all the pain. And this is so bad, I got into this reassignment program to make myself happy and it wasn't working, anymore.

I have not taken a moment to rest and it's my moment to do just that, one I have fought long and hard for, freedom, you know you are free only when you are, you cannot dream about it, My wife always has a snippy rude comment to make, why today?, why that shirt, she hides my makeup, Someone has even taken a razor and slashed some of my nicest dresses and blouses, and I am missing many pairs of shoes? I get a lot of we are busy can't you cancel? We are not busy, just excuses so I don't go out, or I am busy I need the car today, she gets mad when I look at myself in the mirror to check myself after I complete my dressing and grooming, she thinks I am vain, that I just like to look at myself, In conceit, I thought about mirrors, and when I was a child and a teen when I got the chance I would get to see her, (myself) I liked to call it getting a "peek" of myself, it was never a sexual thing or voyeurism, it was just a curios "peek" I was always so excited to see her, I never got to that much, there where weeks months and even years between those ten and twenty minute minutes, I had to look at her and dream for the moment I could be her, imagine yourself a living in a town where there was only one mirror they were very hard to make, the technology was very difficult for us and the material to make them scarce and a man came to each home for a half hour to an hour a day only once, one or two months at a time sometimes you waited a whole year, So that you may see yourself again, just to see what you looked like, you would be as excited as I was, as I awaited my time in front of the mirror to see myself again those fast minutes, I don't really believe I am that beautiful as a woman on the outside, and sometimes I am very paranoid of mirrors now, especially when I am depressed, just like when I see those ugly faces in things like clouds and leaf patterns on trees, I look into a mirror and I see the monster some people in my life say I am becoming Inside is a person for everyone I am in here waiting to share and I have so much love and kindness to offer and all I ask is will you be kind back, nothing more but a smile on your face is all I need, but I just thank god I pass as one, it took years of taking hormones and steroids to get to a point I did not need make up, to go my first ten years in a row without being called sir, unless by accident, or on a phone, but even on phone it's a big improvement, and I understand it's not their fault I don't take it to heart like I used to, I have heard my voice played back "yeck" A phone call that was once a 100 percent failure is now 90-10 I win, I can keep doing better, I just need to keep practicing, I used to have my wife say she was me and listen to the conversation and pass her notes, My youngest daughter has found a boyfriend and is pregnant, he wants to fix our upstairs and move in to help save money to build a salon near a barber shop he owns, the upstairs was once a real nice mother in law type apt, it's a single family home, but the people that lived here before us made the upstairs into a small apt, for their mother, That's why my wife and my oldest daughter wanted to buy this house. I did not want to buy it at all, it needed to much work, and I cannot fix a house I know nothing at all about them, and this is a real fixer upper, What a shack, but the land is the largest lot for a single family home in the town I live in, and I want so bad to move my kids away from that apt. complex were living in. so I said ok, but my oldest daughter and her boyfriend completely destroyed the upstairs, it was so bad you could not use it as an apartment any longer, my two younger daughters took the bedrooms upstairs but closed off the kitchen and bathroom, if I called my insurance company I would have gotten about 40,000 for damages, but it meant my daughter would have been prosecuted also along with her boyfriend for the damage, so I let it go.

She was told to just leave, I was totally ashamed of my daughter, I told my wife before we bought it that this would happen, that they would smash the place to pieces, and neither one of them would ever give you a dime for rent, and I was so right, I love it when I am right But I have never in my life seen a person like my wife warned so many times about things and still make the wrong decision "every time", And she always will. She is going to lose all her children's love someday just like her dad was to her she is to her children, I try everything I can do to break that cycle, but it is very difficult, I feel I will lose in the end, I will always keep trying but I do in vain. Back when the children where sick as small children or scared at night to sleep alone in their beds, They crawled into our room to get into bed with us, If she caught them she kicked them out, they always came to my side of the bed I always let them snuggle with me to comfort them sick or just scared. I did not care sometimes all three of my daughters would sneak in, I would look down at the foot of the bed and see there little heads slowly rise above the head boards, to get a peek at if whether or not we were sleeping, they would sneak into our big king size water bed and all hide at the bottom and sleep. Sometimes it scared the hell out of me, I did not know who it was peeking up at the foot of the bed and staring at me in the dim light, It could have been a stranger robbing the house, it was always a relief to recognize there little faces. they remember that too, they always remember I was the one who cared more when they were sick, I felt there little heads and faces and gave them permission to stay home from school over their mother, when I knew they were not faking or for some reason I knew something bothered them too much to go to school that day, that was certainly a sense I had, I was the more nurturing caring one, and I still am, even my grandchildren come to me first with their aches and pains, It is the nicest feeling in the world to comfort a sick or scared child, I keep hoping my wife will break that cycle passed on to her by her father, but I am not sure, I have taken the sharper edge off but if I was to pass on she would become just like him, And become a reclusive hermit and alone, pick a sibling she likes the most or hopes to bond most with, unfortunately it may be her sister who is worse than her, they would make a perfect couple, it would be sad to see her end up alone with her sister, instead of one of her own children, we had such a bad history with her sister, It actually traumatized me for a long time, I have never been able to forget it. It was when we lived with them in Quincy briefly, very briefly, we shared a two bedroom apartment, we split the rent and utilities and the first couple months it seemed like it was going to work out ok, but things started to make us think there was a problem we bought all the groceries, and for the first three months we got them dinner every night, her sister's boyfriend drank a lot of milk, it was strange, he would drink a gallon at night not a drop left, just himself alone, how does someone drink that much milk? So we buy two gallons and every morning there is about a pint left at the bottom of the second gallon, I did not think a person could even do that, it wasn't that I cared about the milk it was just seemed greedy, and I was amazed he never vomited it back up, he just wanted to pack himself with food like a dog going out to hunt I never saw anyone stuff themselves so much, with milk and food, We fed them every night, now three months straight, and paid rent, And we cooked good meals steaks roasts whole chickens complete home cooked meals, the works, one day he said it's "my treat" tonight, And I am making dinner to show our appreciation for all the meals you have cooked for us, and you're in for a big, big surprise, I wondered all day what I was coming home too, and was I surprised alright, hot dogs and beans, about a five dollar meal for four of us, ha, I just laughed to myself, and said this is not going to work, and then the worst came, a friend of her sister comes to visit, my wife to be is about 5 months pregnant, this is a day off for me during the week as I had to work Saturdays so I got a week day off instead, we had noticed that when we went out things where missing from our room, like cassette tapes, money, change, little pieces of jewelry, clothes, just little things and not a lot but enough to notice, my wife to be then says why is she here? I have things missing every time she is around I don't want her here; you know what she is like why? is she here, what's this?, But her sister defends her friend and says don't let her talk to you like that, go in and punch her, go punch her right in her stomach, go in and kill her baby, that will teach her, go do it, do it. The girl is a girl that has always had a troubled life, lit fires, broke in houses, mother never cared or loved her, She slept in the woods By her house a lot to get away from her drunken abusive parents, but she wasn't that bad, I met her a few times I could tell she could be saved, I hoped someday she will become a real good person if she can meet that person in her life that can bring her to that place she needs to be, to do the right things she really wants to do, I didn't think she would harm a pregnant woman and now at least at that moment I was really hoping not, I was shocked to hear this, I never would have believed it but I was right there in the room listening and heard it myself every word, and no one but my wife knew I was there, it was early in the morning. I just got up out of bed and sat down on a chair, the girl says no way, I am not going to do that, but her sister demands she go in and do it, and for about five minutes beats into this girl like a sergeant to go in and kill go in and kill that baby, the girl was in tears pleading for her to stop! And not to ask her to do something as horrible as that, I am not killing a baby, and the ultimatum came you got thirty seconds or I will do it and say you did! And who do you think they are going to believe me! or a girl with a police record like you, and she started to count down, I just looked at my girlfriend and wife to be, who was just sitting with her face pale anticipating an attack On her and our unborn child, It was as if her sister had some type of jealous rage, Earlier her boyfriend made her get an abortion, and why? I don't know, he was from a rich family, what was he ashamed and afraid of, his rich mother bailed him out of every problem he ever had, One was after we left he was stealing the neighbors tax returns from the mailbox, the whole cover opened with the same key, and everyone's box was exposed, his mistake also was he went to his own bank and cashed them, how stupid is that! He was easily identified, almost went to jail but his parents so being rich got him off, and he was collecting unemployment and going to college, it is a federal offence and they got him with the checks at the same time, he slipped up and said he was a good kid trying to go to college and they said college? Your collecting unemployment you can't, he begged on his hands and knees to the dean to help. Or he would serve six years for that on top of the theft of tax refunds, he got lucky, All he did was play pool at college and it showed he never went to any classes, and his parents, they would have helped with a baby, they were all rich the fathers, father had quite the bank account, and left most of it to just one son, I wonder sometimes if it was his parents decision also to get the abortion, as she was a poor girl from a poor family and they did not want a marriage to bring the two families together, the parents fought a lot about the two of them being together, my wife's sister was actually a very beautiful girl, but it was shocking to hear the rotten mouth on her, what a bully, I then spoke out and said no one will be hitting any one, and it got quiet fast, you could hear a pin drop, Her sister looks in the room and sees me, and says oh yeah, what are you going to do. I said right now I am heading down to where your boyfriend works to have a good talk with him, she said he will kick your ass, I said we will see about that, I don't think he will, and left, his car was at the parking lot where he worked. But when I asked for him they said he did not come in that day, he was in back hiding, I just left, it's what I expected, we moved as soon as we could. And we would not speak to them again for months and wouldn't you know about a year later they follow us, and move to the same complex in a different unit, and act like nothing ever happened, what a funny pair they were, and loaded with money but they came over and stole our towels, wash cloths, forks spoons, wine glasses, plates, we noticed things missing and we couldn't figure it out, till we went over for thanksgiving dinner, I drank wine from my wine glass ate from my plates used my knife's forks and spoons to eat with, I went to wash my hands afterwards and dried my hands with my towels, even the soap was a brand I used, when we left and walked back to our apt, We both said at the same time hey did you notice our stuff was there,? And we just laughed all the way home, rich people, so that's how they stay rich and why would they think we would not notice? Dummies! She is the one who comes Florida to destroy me later when she finds out I have decided to go into a sex reassignment program, and will hold a bitter grudge against me forever it seems, when my wife's gay brother dies we all learn of a trust fund in the family, He wanted his share of his money before he died of the cancer he had in his bladder and now traveled into his kidney, but they were all the holiest of all holy born again Christians, he was an evil sinner and hell was his only destination, and they let him know, by kicking him out of the family in the last moments of his life, and after finding out about the trust fund, his sister my wife's the one from Florida told my oldest daughter she would spend the last dying moments of her life and her last dying breaths making sure that I never in my life ever get one nickel of their families money, Even offered her a very hefty reward to get her into talking her mother into moving to Florida or going alone on a vacation there, so they could take her to their lawyers and doctors to somehow find her unfit to handle her money, and that they would handle her affairs and take care of her for the rest of her life. I don't believe her, she would only abuse her like before, I only hope I can keep the love with her own children alive in case something ever does happen to me, And she doesn't end up down there with those barbarians that's I call them. Her sister says now she is so angelic she can heal you with a touch of her hands and prayer, she would be able to throw away her heart medicine after one session with her, and that scares me, my wife has an enlarged heart now, her output went down to twenty, an output of eighteen and you are dead, she is up to 50-60 now with her medicine and would relapse in a month's time to that low number and die without medicine, to me it's an attempt at murder, although I cannot prove it, I know if she ever went down there alone within six months or so I would get a call there was an accidental drowning or she passed away from heart failure, even a shark or alligator attack would not surprise me, they would not take her to a doctor but to their cult church instead, in fact it would not surprise me at all if it's at church she collapses and dies, all her money would go to these rich people and their children and her own babies would get nothing at all, they would be forgotten as if they never existed, I don't trust them and I never will. They really hate Cynthia and what's worse is, they even hated who I used to be, I was a better person not richer, or had more, just a better person and a better human being, my wife's mother loved me, I was a lot closer to her than my own mother, She did not like her daughters husband at all he was a sneaky little thief always in trouble with the law and very disrespectful to both the parents, neither liked him when my wife's mother had that massive stroke her dad just took over, it was the end of a family who gathered on holidays to spend the day to be together, But when her sister came up from Florida to tell them all I was going to become a woman, they nailed my coffin shut, I never even got to explain myself, I just got the door slammed in my face, and those actions scared my children, People don't realize when they reject me, it comes back a lot harder on my children, I am the one going through it, not them, but they also are the targets of humiliation, which is totally unfair and ruthless and they see their dad once loved and respected by many shamed and ridiculed so publicly, I believe the people and other kids that harass my kids are cowards and bullies, the children out there doing this have learned it from their parents, Most would rather pick on them and not me, why? I am still what I was, a well-trained fighter, I can hit someone in the head so hard there brain would explode, a lot of people that know me from my past know better than to confront me in a dark street, in a corner, they would be in "my world", a world they would leave broken, But I wish not to go there, I have left that behind me. It has given me so much confidence to keep going, even with all the health issues I face now I find strength in my chi, my soul, I take pain and walk it away that would make others weep and crawl, and give in, I have needed that inner strength, without the studies I have completed and still practice when I can, into my busy routine the martial arts and the influence of our Asian culture I have so loved, It would have made my journey 100 times more difficult and scary, I would have been a very frightened timid woman, you will give yourself away especially if your nervous, people first notice your nervous then the next question is why? Why is that person nervous? that's when they start to look more carefully at you and your caught, your caught as a man dressed as a woman right away, And once you give yourself away you feel that fight or flight response, and it gets worse, fear runs through you like high voltage, If so, just relax, take a deep slow breath. If it happens suddenly to you out there, just look away from people, don't make eye contact go to a happy place in your mind. they will stop looking at you, there looking at a nervous person and that's not going to be you, you are now that confident new woman you have chosen to be, you are yourself don't let them steal away an identity you cherish, and want to share, Find your brave face and go forward, every day in my life I give myself my own speeches, I see people that talk to themselves on the street and I know that it's from loneliness for most of them that do it, it seems strange to see someone talking to someone else not there, not so much these days with cell phones but there still out there talking away, they have no phones they are people, all alone forever remembering conversations of the past, maybe a minute or two ago with a friend or stranger or once with their siblings as a child who knows, The reason is that person has spent a long time alone, with no one to talk to, There thoughts of old friends and family, and tragic events in their lives, drop so deep into their soul, their lips move as they think it out, And the deeper they become involved the more they speak with their silent mouths and frightened body language, how do I know this,? I fell deep into loneliness too, so deep I almost never came out, I was starting to get like that myself, but I was aware of it, I also knew if I did not come to a solution one day in my life I would end up in solitude, Sitting on some park bench talking to myself with no one there to listen but my own memories of what I have lost out on, I had fallen that deep into depression, I feel so much for those people when I see them out there, I don't know what happened to them or what in their life lead them to where they gave up and decided there was no hope and why live, And if live at all stay all alone not to be hurt anymore, maybe they unlike me did not prepare or keep a little friend in hiding. in a little safe place someplace in their mind to look for comfort in those days they were scared and alone, And frightened, Or maybe they did and the person inside is all that's left to talk to anymore, they went in to deep and never came back out, It is misery here, out here, when you are alone, and the weather can be so hard on you, it can break down and kill the toughest of any species on the planet, and some of us neglect ourselves and throw ourselves and others we no longer care about out into the cold world to die in the bitter cold all alone, To then stripped naked of your clothing by the others out there trying to survive, as you lie there dying, or dead, This is a choice you make when you decide to just give up and do not want to go on any more, and sometimes I don't think it is a choice I really believe that some people are just too frightened to move, and have become so scared from bullying and harassment in their life that fear drives them out there, not choice, but hate and bigotry has made a world where homeless and starving children and people exist in it, and will always be there as long as all that hate exists, when I walked the streets of California, Oakland and the San Francisco bay area, The homeless where every were the climate was warmer, People slept outside on the lawns of public property like libraries and town hall's, the police came at sunrise to hit each of them on the feet with their Billy club to wake them up for the new day, as if they were the homeless peoples alarm clock, And they all knew where to go to get a breakfast at a local church. If you give up and want to live on the street there it is. you can just fall right into it, when you have nowhere to go and feel all alone it' is' an awful temptation to just let go and give up, but I had to many memories of trying and knowing I should not blame myself, it's not my fault I have this to bare, it should have been addressed very early in my life by my parents, I know they knew and they took so much pride in having that first son, That they refused and denied the reality I was not there son but there daughter, when I sat at that lunch table in high school and that old neighborhood kid revealed to me that when I was about, two, three years old, that five-seven, year old boys came to my house and beat me, I was the boy who wanted to be a girl. I remember those kids as they watched my mother chase me to the bus stop every morning with a hair brush to smack me with if I tried to run back home, It wasn't school I was afraid of, it was them, they just sneered at me as I stood there, and the girls in there little dresses just looked on and watched, no expressions on their faces they just watched, I always felt like I left my body right at that moment, These were maybe my first panic attacks and they plagued me for life, I would get them again in the first grade right after kindergarten when they separated boy girl, boy girl, they did not do that in kindergarten we all used the same restroom, but I remember recess in a big caged area I just leaned against the fence and watched everyone play, I did not know who to play with, recess was always so lonely I would later come out of these panic attacks in the nurses office and my mother would be on her way up to take me home, and the attacks and withdrawing from reality just got worse I even peed myself a few times without even knowing it, or was afraid to use the boys room, how embarrassing, When all those kids laugh at you when you have an accident, like your still a baby, I was scared of getting beaten, not immature, I just could not give in to the bullies and people that hate, giving into myself would be only to the satisfaction to those who hoped I would fail, so I would not, I would keep trying, those people that hated me also where the ones who gave me a lot of my strength and to keep fighting back, They gave me a stubbornness I still have today of not wanting to give up, anything I do I go till I drop, somehow out there would come an answer it was just going out every day and try and look for it, my mother's mother, was my biggest inspiration, to me in my life, as strange as it seems, I would end up not liking my own mother so much, but would find so much strength from her mother, what happens there I cannot explain, she always had good reasoning power, she said she always struggled her entire life when her husband my grandfather got sick and was hospitalized for depression, there were days she took the kids and drove around on buses to keep them warm till they could go someplace for the night to sleep, Never got to rest, or have a break, she told me every day has it's aches and pains, just keep going, I had mine and had to keep going and keep my head up, no matter how bad it gets, and I always heeded her advice. She did it and she did it dragging children along beside her, what strength and courage she had not to abandon them, and she managed to keep all her furniture her husband got from a friend who was a very good cabinet maker of his time during the arts and crafts period of the nineteen hundreds, in a storage bin till she finally got a job and a home and built a family again out of nothing. That is what gave me my drive to keep going and to always care for my own children no matter how hard it was, I worked in places for years some men would only last a week or a few hours in, But my children all of them, never went to bed hungry and without a warm bed to sleep in, and no matter what people will say about me now and what I have decided to do with my life, I was a damn good parent, and a good father, I did my job as a parent and did my best at it and I am still a parent it has never stopped. Only one of my daughters, my oldest who is doing well making six figures a year, has been told to walk out of my life, she says I will destroy her social climbing anyway, I thought I did everything I could not to bring up a child that would be so selfish, but if I think back, when she was a very small child she was so sweet, daddies little girl all the way, I know what I did really hurt and hurt deep, but she was reared by her mother more than me in her early growth, the other two were not, my oldest was so stingy and thrifty her first bag of Halloween candy was still in the fridge the following Halloween, there was a piece or two left, she counted it out to a piece a day, to last her the whole year and she did, I asked her for a piece once she was about 3 years old and off the end of a Hershey bar she snapped of a tiny little crumb to give me, a mouse would have snubbed its nose at such a small morsel, I just laughed, how funny is she to be so cheap, at such a young age, I thought it was something she would grow out of but never did, she like her mother is cheap, you cannot get a nickel off either one of them, but the other two would give you the shirts off their backs, my middle is the sweet kind one she lived here about eight years after my oldest left she married a co-worker a slightly handicapped boy, They get along great, she drives, he cannot get his license I was sad she left and went on their own, my one in the middle was the one that looked the most like me, and is the most generous sincere one of them all, what separates them is she is the quiet one not one to get loud at a party and show off.

but likes to be there, she I believe accepts me more than the others and I feel more comfortable around her than any of my own family, my youngest I feel can accept me now but is influenced by her older sister. And is often frightened by the outcome of things to come that are not the reality just a fear driven fantasy of her paranoid delusional older sister, I wish my oldest daughter would really just get to someone she can talk this out with. That is a reasonable person, what always puzzles me is she has many gay friends male and female and some even bisexual. One of her best friends is a bisexual male and yet I know she has so much hate towards me I feel it from people she is with who should be a little more understanding but there not, so I am assuming she is telling them I am some kind of monster or something to justify her actions, But I cannot dwell on it any longer I had to let her go until she finds peace in herself first then maybe someday me, but I am not expecting that, nor am I waiting and I know I will probably never see her again, my youngest is now here she has moved in with her new boyfriend, And I have just started meeting with my new gender therapist and I tell her how I think it's all going to work out so good but in six months' time and after the baby arrives it's not so good. Just after her boyfriend moved in he decided he would build a salon, for my daughter and he did it for their future, the baby was coming in January and would be a new year's day baby, and I am finding out dad is not the dad I was lead to believe he had done real nice job redoing the upstairs he seemed handy it was now a livable space again. All new bathroom and shower, sink, kitchen all refurbished, he was now renting a large building and remodeling it for the salon, his barber shop was close by my daughter just finished hair dressing school and was good at it, Seemed to want to be in this line of work she almost worked for a model agency posing in wedding dresses got into one catalogue was off to a good start but went to a bar and some girl hit her in the face because she thought my daughter was hitting on her boyfriend, He was hitting on my daughter, she is real hot, and a real looker a Paris Hilton with a "real" beautiful face, so she had a black eye at a very important time, and the photographer could not deal with a girl who was getting in bar room brawl's. Too bad I really feel she had a real career modeling. And missed out on meeting Donald Trump personally, What was funny about this new dad, was his non caring about the birth of his son, He was not waiting or getting ready, more focused on work, when it was time!! He said go wake up your parents they call me dad around here still, see if your dad will drive you! one problem is with my kids calling me dad is they introduce me to their friends as their dad and later have to explain why they saw their dad out dressed as a woman, some I run into leaving the house as they and myself are coming and going, Some I see out in grocery stores or at the mall shopping I see them all over, and they all come over to say hello, it's like half the town knows and the other half does not, and the two worlds are going to collide soon and when they do it's going to be like coming out again all over, I am not looking forward to it, and this should never have happened in the first place, but it has, I was out of work on SSI disability, so I am not really dressing as much as I should be and a lot of it is, my own fault, I am in street clothes more and in the house or at home, I don't feel well often so I stay in, I am either in too much pain or fatigued from my auto immune I have a sleep disorder, I have had since high school and rarely sleep, so dressing up nice has slowed down just doctor appointments, Or anything that I have to go in and say yes I am Cynthia in a professional way of any sort, also the hormones and my hair length has made my appearance very feminine I pass well without make up, I have become very feminized it's been ten years since I have been call sir except maybe by someone who can recognize a transgender person, Either they know one or they see them at clubs they hang out at, or I just slip up and that damn low voice sneaks out and I get some wise guy that wants to make an office joke out of me. In fact that happened to me at a very bad time in my life dealing with severe depression. Not more than a year ago I went to get dental work done at a teaching school the prices are good and for a root canal you get a real intern, a doctor, I signed in as Cynthia I wore a t-shirt no makeup, An early morning quick dentist appointment, I have a bra on I have my own breasts now a C cup I am very happy with them, at my age of 56 they are still firm and perky, but I notice the woman who signed me in keeps peeking over the desk at me. In-fact I got a little creeped out and moved my seat, but thought nothing of it, though she still peered over the counter at me, then I was called in, was treated very good there by everyone I interacted with and then at the end I had to pay, I had made a money order out for the amount they told me on the phone but it was a little over ten dollars more than it need to be So I made the money order out to high, So I asked do I get change from a money order? And the woman that signed me in said hold on now there "SIR" let me check that, for you "SIR" and then a loud hey do I give "HIM" change back if "HE" gives me a money order. I am shocked I look at her and say it's not sir it's "miss', my name is Cynthia! another woman behind the counter says no "miss" we have to mail it to you, then real loud I hear, well there you go "SIR" they're going to mail it to you, anything else we can do for you "MISTER" I look and people are stopped and looking at me, and looking at her, I was so embarrassed I just left, I was shocked! And a little scared what was she doing that for? what if someone who thought killing someone like me and you do the world a favor was standing next to me and followed me out and shot me dead in the street, and a woman standing beside me was just in the ladies room with me, I emailed the schools human recourse dept., the following day to let them know how I was treated. and that I was in fact a transgender woman and I believe she picked up on it and harassed me in front of a group of people, And had embarrassed me terribly and maybe others around me, (especially the woman beside me who had just came out of the ladies room with me) I did not tell them that part, but I felt bad for that woman she may have gotten scared or embarrassed herself, There response was very good! and they all apologized to me it was nice to get that support back and a promise no one else like me would ever have to go through that again there, and I hope it opened that door to others so they are not ever treated that way if they should go there to get a bad tooth fixed, I got that behind me with the help of the people in the administration of the school and a sincere apology from the dean of the university and a kind hearted follow up, from them all, I am doing well and moving forward, I only hope that woman is getting help and was never punished. just lead in the right direction, she was a black woman too and you would think they would be a little more sensitive to discrimination, but the world is color blind more than I thought, my new therapist was a nice soft easy woman to talk to, the first time I meet her it took a long time to find her, I was in a panic from getting lost, The first time I tried I never made it, I got so lost, it was the day Michael Jackson died, but we had some nice talks together, my last visit I left there thinking everything was ok at home but I was so wrong it went so bad, all of a sudden I was getting snapped at for putting on a woman's coat or blouse, I was getting asked why are you wearing that you don't have to work anymore, you don't have to wear those clothes, and this, is my wife, talking to me, Who has seen me a thousand times is now asking why? And I hear that my daughters new boyfriend wasn't told yet, but I was surprised, I know he knew, I knew I was being lied to, my oldest was coming to the house saying the only reason he is here, is to catch you in a dress, so he can take custody of the baby he doesn't want his son around someone like you. I said he already knows, he is playing games he can't take away a baby for that, she said just watch, they got money and they want that baby boy, all to themselves, so I am shocked, but I still don't' believe it, his ex-best friend was my daughters ex-husband, And he knew, he saw me all the time, His family did not want him to stay married to my daughter because they did not want someone like me in there family, and they made her life hell, and now again, why did she even date this guy knowing all this, and then I find out he is bi-polar and won't take medicine, the nice peaceful quiet of the upstairs breaks he has lost his manners let's say, He starts out louder each day testing our limits, walks the floors all night moves furniture constantly all night rearranging the rooms, starts fighting with my daughter and won't let her out to visit friends or let them visit, The salon was not just a place for her to work, it was a prison he was building around her so he could watch every move she made, A real control freak and I am finding out my daughter is terrified of him, talking to her everyday seems useless, but I do anyway I am not giving up till she will get him out of her life and start a new one, someday she will get away and be free of him, she is almost there but she has to be careful, he may just snap and hurt her real bad maybe even kill her, With all this going on and me being threatened with the baby I have also helped my daughter raise, I have probably been the closet one to him since he was born, My daughter wanted me right up there with her all the time helping, what an awesome feeling that spite it all, my own daughter knew I was that good a parent and not an evil monster and of all the people around her she chose me to help her with her new tiny infant, it was such a blessing to me she will never know, and how happy that made me that she chose me over her own mother, I am being careful for my daughter as what I hear upstairs is not good, the fighting was bad, I asked her what she wanted me to do. but she wanted to take care of it herself, there is that I will take care of it myself answer I got from her older sister, it took a violent ending to stop that one, I hope that this ends a lot better, it would be best if he just became the dad he should be, the restraints on me are getting hard I am so glad I have been in touch with my friend, I had always and still loved so, and could still talk about anything, anything at all, she is just so special a real wonderful woman and a real loyal friend, I had always had that place specially held in my heart for ever for her, that one you only find once, I saw her often, sometimes for me a little too much, I never lost any of the feelings I had, they are all still here. like a jewel in a watch keeping my heart beating, And it was a sad feeling to always still feel alone and again to see her Especially now at a time all this was going on, it was a lot for me to take in, emotionally I was just breaking apart and my family was also, I got into a very depressed coma like state I could not get away from and slowly slid further into, and just stayed in it, I smiled on the outside but I drifted off all day and night with death fantasies again and real heavy, That warm, warm blanket again, starting to plan suicides again and it was just worse at home my was wife hiding some of my makeup and started hiding other things, and when I confronted her she denied it, but later said she was trying to keep the peace, she said there going to take the baby, If he sees you dressed as a woman, he is taken the baby and taking full custody of it and I would never see it again, and that is that. I say that's not possible and then it's just a fight every day to go out and I am not backing down, and then I still got my oldest one stopping by. here and there taking her shots at me, and I think it makes her feel good she can come back here and find a way to get at me again and they are using a baby against me! of all things to use, another baby, this time one I have been with since an infant, Just days old I was holding him and rubbing his little back to comfort him and burp him out, he felt like my own little baby, and there telling me now that if he sees me in makeup or any woman's clothing he will stop at nothing to take his son away from anyone like me, his son was not to be exposed to some freak like me, but I know myself that he cannot do that I went through this before I already had DSS at my house before, They never found anything to investigate on me with they always closed my cases, I remember the very first time they came a neighbor who was always drunk and my wife and I fought with, There daughter was a bad influence on ours, called on us, said we were beating our kids when they checked my kids my oldest had a bruise, I knew nothing of it but years later found out her uncle was over, and my oldest was in the house mouthing off to her mother Her uncle was so shocked at her language and the way he treated his sister he just grabbed a toy plastic bat chased her outside and smacked her on the behind, and not to beat her just a bap, and the neighbor saw him and reported him, But she told them I did it, she said I was beating my kids with a baseball bat, they closed the case after a few visits, I told them if they want to come to my house and tell me how to raise my children then I will just leave, and you can stay here full time and raise them for me, the neighbor died a few years later after, from alcohol poisoning, people like her that abuse child services and tie them up on needless cases while real abuse is out there, should get penalties for such abuse to the system once they were useful a couple lived there with a little girl and the father always had a case of beer in his arms and an open can, and two or three for the weekend, sometimes we see them leave without their child we assumed she was with a babysitter or her grandparents, but she was at home locked in her closet. They set up a little table and chair made a little bed for her and left food then locked her in for the weekend and took off, they got caught, and their daughter was taking away from them. Now that was a time DSS was useful. and I was glad they came to help, what if there was a fire or she choked on a sandwich, but they should never be used to just harass someone for revenge and hate, and for pranks, It's horrible to have these people come into your private lives and threaten you with the taking of your children if you don't cooperate, on the call of a drunken prankster, Who is herself abusing her own children, but it's over, only now it's with my youngest daughter and her boyfriend and him making these threats, I feel like my own baby is being taken from me, I have helped raise him since he has been home, I have changed him and cleaned him up more than his mother and my wife and his dad all together and have watched him grow and change from an infant to a toddler even his fist steps I was there, it is no different than if I was a woman locked in a prison, Surrounded by angry guards who were coming to take my baby away and give it to someone who would never love it as much as me, and no matter how many times I could explain it to them I know I can never reach them, I was there, not his dad, me, and they are now going to just snatch him away and never let me see him again, I am just deep in a depressed coma, I have not seen my gender therapist for a while now, I have been seeing my other therapist for my depression and anxieties, I don't know how this poor woman can handle what I come in and tell her some days, I see her once every week but I had quit my depression medicine a year ago.

it was aggravating my restless leg syndrome, and not really working to well, the head doctor at the clinic had cancelled me three times in a row, because she was too busy and passed me off to someone else and I got hurt, I knew her more than twenty years, I did not want to suddenly change and start over, I really felt rejected and had lost another friend, all my hormones where off there scales I had not adjusted to the male hormone block yet the dose was not big enough. and because of my age I have to take less of the female hormones to prevent blood clots and strokes, and the male hormone block is a little hard on my stomach so I am super PMS 'n bad on top of being in such a depressed coma, I also am still keeping in touch with my friend we email a lot and I get to visit once and a while, I just sneak out when I can, seeing someone you once felt that strongly for is very difficult and those feelings can come right back and grab a hold of you, and you know so much has changed that even if you wanted so bad to have her back the possibilities are just about non existing you don't even hope you just know, and you know you will only hurt yourself more trying, she knows how I feel I tell her everything in my life and in my heart, she is still the only person in the world I can share anything with, and she is as beautiful as ever, She is not well she is slightly crippled with rheumatoid arthritis but I don't care it makes me want to care even more for her. I cannot bare to see her in pain, I feel her pain as I feel my own, I feel like I am still connected at the soul with her and it never and will never be disconnected just like I thought, and I am happy it never did, she has really come to accept me and love me as Cynthia and accepts her more than anyone else I have known, But except a few, I know she feels the same, she still loves me as much as before and I know that she knows how important it is that I continue on through my journey. To become the complete woman I am to be. And she would never stop me or cause me to hesitate one step, in anyway, as if she knows what's best for me, and wants to me continue on even if it meant we would never be together again as a couple or embrace again once more, what a loving sacrifice she has given to me, she needs a man in her life, a real good man, not me, not a woman, I know her needs, and I know she wants and needs a man in her life, no matter how hard I would try I would not make it, I could break my own heart trying, but I could never break hers, I wondered what it would be like to stop now and come back to being a man again. Right now if I had to, how would that be? it could happen, I wonder what would happen if a major war broke out and medicines where no longer available and I would have to change back, First of all I most likely would not live long without nitro stats I would have a heart attack soon within days or weeks after, But not just that, to stop and decide I want to just stop I can no longer go on, it's just too painful to continue, I am hurting to many people, it would be very hard, not so much the physical change but the emotional change I have been through, I have experienced 20 years of my life nurturing my female side into becoming a woman and not just the physical but the emotional side and the experiences I have had of being one, If I think it was hard as a teen growing up, it would be one hundred times harder to live with that woman in a man's body feeling I would have again, it would feel like a shell is growing around me closing me up inside like a caterpillar that went into its cocoon and made it too thick to break out, only my legs and arms stick out and my eyes pop through I would look and feel like a Mr. potato head running around in circles, always carrying this heavy weight on my back, just an ugly little bug, hoping somebody will step on me and put me out of my misery. The butterfly would be trapped inside forever, it would never be able to break out of its little prison and fly free and show it's beautiful wings. I would have that feeling for the rest of my life, if the world where different and men could show more feelings it would be great, but not enough, I thought of life without mirrors, how would I know what I looked like without one as like in the beginning of the book I used a chair to expose myself to the reader to be out there naked not hidden under blankets and silk sheets. If I would follow my instincts and do things I like doing I would be with the ones I feel I associate with, I would want to be with woman, I would want to help with children and make sure they are fed and clean, but they would see me as a male if I had this male body and drag me away, Tell me what I do is wrong. and that I have to be with the men, I am one of them not a woman, and only looking at each other without clothes would tell me, they are right, if we were all covered up and looked the same then it would be confusing and I believe that many people in that situation would be, Rules should be made, like we have now, men cannot in this society appear to look like a woman and it makes sense, I am not trying to put every man in a dress, if we were all the same we would panic, but for someone like me in this world and in the reality of my life for me to feel I am a complete person I have a need to look who I feel like I am and that is a woman. I cannot fit myself in this world any other way with my personality the part of my identity that makes up part of my brain that is my "self" I wake up every day I am that same person living in the same house, same pets, same children, I know every day who I am, and I can't change that, I never have been able to, unless I had a lobotomy, I asked one time if I could have that piece of my brain taken out that tells me what sex I am, so I could be normal, so far they say no. It would make it all easier if they could go in with a scalpel and uncross those wires, but what would I be, I would have to build a complete new identity again, It would be like putting another person inside my body, and adapting it to be my life, So many pages of my life would be blank I would recognize a lot of people, but not know who they are, or places I have been, just a lot of feelings I have been here before, myself as it is, my being as it is, will remain and be happy in this world, only in the female body, it is the safest most comfortable place to be, that's what I feel most as a woman, I feel safe and comfortable in my role, it fit's. it's not a mask, or a costume or a phony name I made up for the night, It's me and if I was to be a man and have the personality I have, sure I would be ok, I would have some friends who would say what a nice sensitive guy or what a sweet one, is he gay? I would be more alone as a man than I would be as a man trying to become a woman, I already know my several attempts to find a woman and build a relationship never got past the too gentle touch by my own hands, and I cannot change that, it's me, I cannot stop, the people around me that truly love me will release me into womanhood and not hold me back. The ones who don't love me will hold me back as long as they can, and I have so many holding me back at this moment that I want to just an end all this pain, I felt a little crush from that old flame of love again to. I did not think I would have that feeling again, so strong for someone. But it was her she is just special I cannot let myself fall in love with her again, I know what we have had before and I know the feeling in my heart and exactly where it is so I can watch it and be careful that I don't lose control of it, and I know that I must keep going and not break any more hearts or hurt anyone except myself, I would only sacrifice myself, I would only hurt myself first before others, suicide was becoming a real option once more, my wife's father died and she is now going to inherit a little money, and her sister now turns up the heat, she has been still trying to get my wife down to Florida so she can get control of her life and money. My kids tell me of a botched plan to get her to the airport and that a ticket was there waiting, All they needed was a driver, they called all my kids to see who would do it, they were told that they were doing this to help, and that I! There dad was just going to take all their moms money, and spend it on sex change surgery and they would see that I didn't and that they would reward my kids for their help. And that I was evil, the devil has possessed me, but my kids did not give in they would not drive her, the plan fell through, I was not told yet, also they came to the house, I did not see them I did not want to I left for the day, But they tried to get her to go with them to the airport and back to Florida with them, but she would not go, she told them her children and grandchildren need her and they told her none of her own children love or care about her at all, And to come with them, she will have everything she wants, what evil monsters to not only try to take my wife from me but to take a mother from her own children and grandchildren, so they can have her money to give to their children and their grandchildren and mine would be left out in the cold and forgotten, they would never help one of our children ever, it is all lies by evil cult worshippers, I was thinking I should try a new anti-depressant to help get me out of this dark place, I was getting to a point where I was so depressed when I looked at clouds I saw scary faces in them and hideous monsters, not little cars or houses, horses, doggies, flowers, this was the start of deep depression, I have gotten like this before I was looking at a bouquet of roses with baby's breath mixed in the arrangement it should be beautiful to look at, but it turned ugly, little monsters and mean faces peered through the shapes of the tiny leaves, flowers and shadows. Everything outside in the spring had no beauty, it all looked flat, and dull, two dimensional, and I could not look long at anything, the human brain has a way of seeing faces in things and mine was seeing the worse of them, And it was again, I was still a little unwilling I really wanted to die, taking an antidepressant may make me not want to, It was my therapist for depression who got me to go back on them and my sweet little friends little voice of wisdom I try so hard to listen to and need so much, but what really made me go back on them was when telling my therapist some of my death fantasies and how they had become so poetic, she turned to adjust a blind, so she had said, but she turned to cry, and I saw a few tears fall from her eyes, genuine ones to, and it broke me right there I could not hurt another person, I was caught up in wanting to stop my own pain I forgot about the others of people who really do care and that brought feelings back in me I had lost, so I went back on medicine it worked for a few weeks but once I got through the sample pack and the dose got high, it back fired, it did the opposite, it made me worse, but before I went down real hard with depression, I got out one day with my friend and we went to a cook out I changed at her house, she had a date, and was so excited and I for her also, She was going to meet him there, I did not mind at all I was happy she would have a man in her life, I was never jealous at all, Although I loved her so much, I knew it was just better to leave it alone, and just be good friends as woman, it was to me so wonderful just to be loved by someone as myself, and especially to have her as my girlfriend as a woman, I could not ask for more, It was going to be fun her daughter was there and I saw her looking at me with a comfortable smile on her face, she made me feel very relaxed I looked at her and said I just feel right, I had a nice black flowered pattern dress that almost came to my feet and nice shoes, of course, and I noticed she looked at them she just smiled as she took me all in, she said you look good, you must have known a long time you were like this? I said I have known since I can remember, never in my life feeling any different it has been a life time to get here, I really mean it when I say I feel right, her daughter also at one time did something for me she never ever at the time realized how much kind of an act she had done, I had gone to visit for a moment and her baby daughter ran about the house playing without any clothes on that day, just a crazy day for a mother, And when I knocked at the door, she welcomed me in, she did not slam the door shut on me and say come back later, I'm busy. Or close it and talk through a crack in the door, and I would have understood, it would have been ok, I understand parents and their children, I had my own, and not have been hurt, while back at home my own family was scaring me, and surrounding me like viscous attack dogs threatening to take my baby away and making me feel like I was a monster, this kind woman opened the door up and let me in, she will never know at that time in my life how much she did for me then, That simple little act of kindness at a time when I needed it so much, was a lifetime of love, in a moment, a twinkling of an eye, it is so easy to love and we don't even know when we do sometimes, and I will remember her forever for that, when you receive so little a taste of something sweet in your life and do not get much of it and expect it no more, You cherish that moment of sweetness on your lips forever, so not to forget that should another come along it will bring you back there for a moment of feeling someone loved you once more, and especially when you feel so alone, for so long a time and hope again someone will be kind even once more, It helps so much keep you in a good direction, and those special people if you find them somewhere in your life keep them, don't let go of them, even if they move far away, always remember them, they will be there when you need them, even though they may be a thousand miles away, Off we went to the party, all dressed nice and for the first time in so long out as a woman and two girls out to have fun, I don't get a lot of those, work was always a joy, every day was like this, I loved going to work just for the companionship of woman, and to dress as one of them and be in there world, it took a lot of my disabilities and at their peaks and to be hit more than with one at a time to get me so sick I could not work anymore, This day out was going to be so much fun and like being alive again, But back at home my wife had called the clinic and said I went crazy and was in the house abusing her. and then left, they tried to call back to verify her story to make sure it's not a prank, but I have call block and the new operator could not get through, there is a special number the caller has to use to get through most know it, this poor new girl almost got fired, I told my youngest daughter I would be gone for the day but not my wife, she would have found some lame excuse to keep me in, she never wants to do much, except go for walks at a park that just hurts my back so much every time we go, and she gets drastic to the point she will block the car in the driveway, and make a scene outside screaming to get attention, and possibly the police, she is a handful. And wants to control everything I do, I to married a control freak, but I fight back, it is a constant struggle, she is like a thief in a hotel, turning every doorknob looking for one unlocked a way in. to get you, I watch her every day and get her off me, as soon as she tries to get in control, it is the time I am dominate and have to be, and will be, and I don't like it, It is another area we lost touch, I do not like that I want everything mutual, especially when it came to me putting on a dress and going out, She acts like it's a big deal and I am putting her out of her way, when to me it's a very special moment, and this is why I still do not believe she loves me and that means "me as a woman", she wants her man back, but he is not coming back, he was never here, and what little she had, and could have made a wonderful spouse of she rejected him when she rejected who I was really inside, and I have worn dresses so many times why does it still bother her, and why does putting on makeup upset her or anyone, I look like a woman either way, what's wrong with a little extra grooming, It's just caring for myself, everyone needs to, it's important to take care of yourself, It's the first step to loving yourself, When I go to see my therapist she wants me to explain myself, the switchboard rang off the wall all day, and if they had got a return call to the house and my wife repeated what she said to the operator, they may have sent the police out to look for me, I was shocked, but not surprised she would go to that length to control my cross dressing or just to go out by myself to think and be alone, and it's not cross dressing for me anymore I am a woman I have been legally female twenty years now, and it gives me a double identity feel to say I am cross dressing now, although in my life I did feel like I was in a battle with two personalities and only one could win. Cynthia and I had a song, it was Helen Reddi's me and you against the world, but I am not two, just one cut up by everyone else that wants a piece of me to fill their needs, and not my own any more. what more is there but the table, the laws have changed, I am legally a woman now, no one should be bothering me about what and when I wear anything, and taking care of ourselves is important, We all need that, with the boyfriend of my daughter still at the house making his threats, not to me just my daughter who tells her oldest sister who fuels the fire saying I was the reason they took her son, when it was a restraining order on her boyfriend issue not me, He was actually terrorizing everyone in there, my home was almost under siege except me I was not afraid of him, but I could not get anyone in the home relaxed, And with help with any of this, I just fell deeper into depression, the battle to be myself, just to put on a blouse and eyeliner was a battle, I was adjusting in hormone changes like a super PMS along with the depression medicine that back fired and what they were doing to me at home, It was a perfect storm for a suicide and I got deep into a fantasy for the first time so deep I got poetic with my thoughts it all started to come together like it was going to happen I even started to plan and had a place a time and a method, I just needed to have all three together in one place, I was going to buy a white candle and bring it with me to a place near where I live, a white lit candle is a symbol of love, I was in stores looking at the ones I wanted to buy, some are very expensive when you get ceremonial candles, and I was bringing the method, I had decided on an overdose of Benadryl, I had just read an article it was the new choice woman where using to commit suicide with, I liked that it was a woman's choice, and I liked that I wanted to use a womans method, also plan 2, I had m-98 fireworks, I wanted to put three in my mouth and wrap duct tape around my mouth and blow my head off, I was afraid if I died they would put me in a three piece suit and bury me, and put my old name in the paper and no one who knew Cynthia would know I was gone and could say goodbye, so if I blew my head off there would be no daddy to kiss good bye, and they would have to close my coffin, but that was not what I really wanted, the Benadryl woman s choice I was still was interested in. I would take enough to just about pass out then take the lethal dose, my lit candle I was to blow out before I fell to sleep, and leave a note, just a small one, like me so small in this big lonely world, that read this white candle lit is a symbol of love and the candle died out from not anyone caring about it, I never in my life thought of a note, or leaving one behind, I thought I would always dress as a woman and when they found me it would explain enough, but for the first time ever. all the years I thought out suicide, this time I had a note to leave behind, and I knew I meant it, I could not stay any longer, with no love at home, the threat of my baby being taken from me, my heart broken, I was headed to my grave or a hospital, I was warning my therapist, I was getting deep and may need to check into a hospital, and I was serious, I was always afraid I would not succeed and do brain damage like many do and only make things worse, I did fail! Twice! As a teen, failing scared me! Or I really had to make sure I did not and be ready to go face god, I cried for days nonstop I hid from everyone, tears start to stop falling after a few days they kind of dry up and they slow down not falling that much but they were there just at the cusp of the wave waiting to fall out of the eye to slide away and die, like I want too, I told everyone I was sick I stayed in bed and hid in my blankets as much as I could, the only reason I had decided to take any anti depression medicine was the one day with my therapist as I explained my candle and note, and it hurt me so to hurt another, and one as special like herself, I really had a lot of feeling for her more than just a friend and I have just hurt her, again I was feeling love for others, that was a good sign no one saw me crying that I knew of, I told my middle age daughter I was not well and I may have to go into the hospital, I trusted her the most, I told her I had to break free or I could not go on, news got to my oldest daughter that I wanted to come back out again regardless of any of the consequences and dress everyday whenever I just felt like it, no reason at all, I just wanted to, I had to email in everyday to the clinic, To let my therapist know I am ok my oldest daughter started to harass me again blaming me that her mother has not got her inheritance yet because her family hates me so much and was brewing trouble with her siblings, she told my youngest daughter the state took her baby away because of me and her boyfriend will soon get his son away from her, and it would be my fault, if I come back out, I reassured her it was a restraining order issue with her violent boyfriend and not me. It can be proven in time, but she was scared, her boyfriend had her frightened and so didn't my oldest daughter, I could do nothing to reassure her, I was nearing the end, I arranged a meeting with my wife and I with my therapist for depression, my wife talked the most, it went ok but later my wife said she felt gained up on, but my wife did all the talking I listened, no one gained up, we knew That was not going to work, my wife gets a call, It's her therapist from the clinic, she had cancelled and they wanted her up there to talk to her, because not only am I a transgender woman but an elderly handicapped person and she knows it, I should not be scared frightened or harassed either way in my own home for any reason, I hear her trying to explain herself and being asked who was bothering Cynthia at home, my oldest daughters name kept popping up, and she is told and I am told that I am not to come to the clinic without woman's clothes on or I cannot come at all, I am excited to hear this, it was an intervention at my home I needed so bad, I can get dressed now without a fight, a new doctor I meet with tries a new medicine, Remeron it helps me sleep but still not getting me right, it's a medicine used for people very depressed, my oldest daughter found out I was dressing and going out again, she had got laid off work and was at home, to cause me trouble, I was at an appointment, she came to the house and was going to attack me when I arrived home, she told her mother and she went and got a big shovel, and hid so when I came home and around the corner to the door she was going surprise me and try to beat me to death with it, My wife told her to leave and informed the police, my daughter did not come back she may have tried to but saw the police cars at the house, I got nasty emails from her, what horrible language, you would swear the devil himself was spewing out his anger at you, so I just said we have to say goodbye to each other now, if this is how you still feel, I will not change, I am who I am now forever, I will not ever change back, that person is gone, and I said goodbye, what a relief that was, she was gone, a demon in my life was gone. I got some more real nasty disgusting emails from her I wrote back to tell her to stop and she should just thank me for raising her kid for her while all she did was party all weekend, And would not be successful if I was not there for her to raise her child she abandoned, and she went to the police station to try and get me in trouble, for what I don't know, her emails would have got her committed, And soon another bad fight broke out upstairs with my daughter and her control freak boyfriend, he came and stayed upstairs with her, they did not date or go out, she just worked at his salon that is the only way she gets money for the baby, The little piece of dirt will not pay child support she has to work for it and if there are no customers tuff luck, lucky she is here and she has me to help or she would really be in trouble. he says he does not have to pay any child support or help with anything at all with money, because he built a salon, He has never even bought a box of diapers and he came there just to keep her a prisoner, She cannot go out talk to her friends, watch on television what she likes, he watches jersey shore and acts like all those people, they treat each other like trash, and that's how he treats my daughter just like she is trash, and she could get any man in town, in a second, and he knows it, he is a five foot ugly little troll with no self-esteem and hates woman, he treats woman like dogs, even his own mother is abused by him, his father walked out when he was about six years old, he never had a male figure to discipline him and teach him to respect people especially woman, He treats them like trash, I sometimes really believe he is a gay man in denial and will one day have a boyfriend.

A male lover, like I was once accused of by that therapist in Quincy as a teen, But only, I adore woman, and would only treat one like I would want to be treated myself as one, that's the first difference, and many more between what I would call a gay man and a woman trapped in a man's body. A fight happens at around, one AM, and as I am just waking up police are at the door. My wife called them and I know she would not have called unless she heard something that really scared her, she hates to involve the police, and my wife becomes so scared for her own safety blocks our entrance downstairs with chairs and the police cannot get in to talk to me, and I am very upset, my wife is hysterical and yelling at the police, interfering with their whole investigation and they ask my daughter what happened but she is too scared of this man to say anything, and from what they see from the way my wife is acting they feel sorry for "HIM" and we look like we are the white trash that the boyfriend is calling us when he talks to the police, And they help him leave, and comfort him for having such a bad night, but I go to the police station in the next afternoon to meet with the shift field commander and explain how he has had all the woman in the home under siege and has them all frightened at the house and is violent, and has smashed my doors to get in to get at my daughter, and that's why the mother acted the way she did and interfered, But I told him if they ever come to my house again for a domestic and anyone at all interferes with the police and distracts them I don't care who it is, I want them restrained or arrested if needed, I said I want you in there to get your job done he has kicked our doors in many times to get in and chase her down to beat her, but no one can do anything until she gets the courage to tell someone, I tell her every day to get strong and stop being afraid, I have even offered his head on a plate but she is reluctant, I would easily slip into the night and find him alone and handle justice for my daughter if it needs to be, and not that I want to be a man and do it a man's way, but I will still use the skills I have and knowledge to protect anyone I love, who cannot protect themselves, especially my own, she is a woman caught up in that viscous cycle of abuse, but this time the boyfriend is gone and won't be back, I will put the restraining order on him myself if he ever comes here again and displays any use of anger to get what he wants and now that he is gone and my older daughter along with him and I am getting some sleep and finally my freedom back the sunshine is coming in through the windows to plant new life, But I still need something else to get out of this dream like state I am in, it tires me so and makes me weak and helpless still. I still need to add something to this medicine or try another, I decided to keep trying, For the few people I know really care about me, I did not want to do this for myself to much anymore I am tired and have had enough abuse and so tired of tears that hurt, I like the ones that feel good to release. I am giving a medicine to take in the morning when I wake up called Dexedrine, given to patients with ADH, The kids in school with ADD got all the attention because they were loud and disruptive kids, While sad and depressed kids like me quiet alone in the corner got forgotten and just pushed ahead, but really left behind, I tried it the first few days it was already working my head was getting clear, it felt like I woke up from a bad dream and remembered everything. Or was a real bad drunk at a party and was so embarrassed afterwards and felt I had to apologize to everyone I scared or hurt, and I started to think about my wonderful kind little friend again and if I hurt her in any way at all or scared her I would never forgive myself I cannot harm this one ever, and was suddenly taken off my feet as I felt an overwhelming feeling of sadness and grief, like never before, she was my best friend, my first real true love, and a little warm candle I kept lit in my heart, and I cried so hard, even more than before I could not stop myself, Not at all, I thought it was my old crush returning but no, it could not be that, I had that happen over a month ago, and when I felt it grow, and start wanting her again I backed away, I even told her I was having my old feelings coming back, I had seen her a little too much and was at her home doing little things around her apartment for her fixing little things and started to crush out, But I knew what that felt like and this was not that this was much more intense, this was different and new, and very powerful it was all I could feel I could not even hear anything around me, and felt I was going to just float away but I felt way to heavy, and very weak, and pictures of her flashed through my head and opening emails made me shake a little, I suddenly realized what was happening to me and it was so amazing, I wish at that moment I had a vile with a cover so that when I had cried those moments I could have poured the tears I cried into a little bottle and saved them, and put them away in a real little jewelry box to treasure forever, I had fallen in love again, but this time I was a woman, I had fallen in love as a "woman," and not a crush real love, way inside, a real heavy feeling as if the earth was taking me into it deepest parts, my first love I had, that one and only time, I always thought that if I fell in love with her again I would know it, and sense it creeping up on me in daily thoughts as they grew, along with the love replanted, I know her feeling, I can put my finger right on my heart when I think of her and point to where I feel her, it's always there, But this was so different it came right in through the side door and took me completely by surprise, and I never in my life time ever enjoyed every tear that fell from my eyes as much as I did then, when I realized why I was crying, and what happy tears they were, those one you want, it was the most amazing feeling I ever had I had fallen in love as a "woman", That little candle I always kept lit for her it separated into two separate pieces and lit up inside me like the sun itself and filled me with feelings and emotions I never knew existed, and what was so amazing afterwards I had feelings, nice ones not all the sad depressed ones for the last thirty years real ones like everyone else, what a change, I had control again of my life, My head was on straight I was dressed as I should be, The end of a long battle that finally ended and I came out winning, And I finally had that chance again to look at myself and not be scared and feel lonely, More than a peek at myself, This is forever, I was getting treated without any more hostility I was free again, out of my box, and I was never going to hide myself away like that again ever, I am free and not just dreaming, I feel it! and I thought of my little box and what I would do with it, it was with me so long now, saving me all those times I needed a place to go and find comfort when I was scared and lonely, Would it just fade away into my memories? or would I just have an old jewelry box to remember myself trapped in, this was a real dilemma for me, that little safe place I had all my life, I still felt attached to it. I felt I could not let it go, I have so many memories of being safe and having a safe place to grow, and it came to me that I had always felt that I only fell in love once in my life, but now I have fallen in love twice, once as a man and now again as a woman. What a wonderful experience that was for me, and the two are separate feelings and emotions and they are very different from each other. Falling in love as a man and falling in love as a woman were two very amazing emotions to have a chance to experience, and you would only know if you were me! And did what I have done, I decided, at that moment. I would take my two most precious memories that I have of falling in love, And put them in my little special box and place it in my "heart" forever, And those days I am scared lonely and frightened and I know many of those days will still come, I still have my little box to go to and a place to go off and explore and grow together with my new feelings and emotions and dreams and hopes, just like before, only this time I am free, not locked inside, the time I spend there now will be times of pleasure and comfort and memories to help me grow to be the woman I was born to become, I have found that as I write this book, it has the same quality, As I write each draft and go back over it and make it better each time before it is ready to be given to anyone to read, that the book grows with me and I grow with the book, My youngest daughter a hair dresser colored my hair back to blonde it was black for a long time, like my mother was, but my grandmother was a blonde woman but I am more blonde naturally anyway, I wanted a change when I first went out and now again like a rebirth of myself, a whole new woman appears before me in that mirror that is me, That beautiful woman I have so wanted to share with everyone has arrived, this time she is staying here I am not going back, I am out of my box and I am standing right here in front of you. The love inside that I had I had pushed it away myself, and let others let me but I am not any more, I have made that last important step I needed and I felt it for the first time ever in so long, A feeling I held frozen suspended in time was love, And now I loved myself, And whether or not anyone else will or not it won't matter unless I do first, I have made it, I have become a woman, I am more alive than ever before, I have all new feelings and emotions that I never knew I had and I know that I have only just touched the surface and I have many new emotions and adventures to explore all I needed was someone special who I knew loved me to take my heart by the hand and give it that little push it needed to come back to life, I am thankful for the few people in my life that guided me through this and gave the "hope" I saved for so, so long, a chance to become a reality, And the one special person I embraced so long ago and loved so much, and always will love! the little candle I kept lit and warm in my heart, I would never let go cold or give up on came and saved me, when it had grown into its new form, along with all the wonderful feelings of what it really feels like to be a woman, I feel I have made it, I told her once long ago someday I would write a book and I always felt she was special to me. And someday I would find a way to write a wonderful love story in the end, but I never imagined it would be here in this book like this, but I am really not to surprised, that love had made me the woman I am today and I got it from her, and I will continue to keep growing with the two wonderful little treasures she gave me, I will keep them in my heart forever, two little candles lit now forever to grow and keep me warm, thank you

Sincerely with love
and love always, forever
Cynthia Marie